men's HEALTH
HANDBOOK

Dr Michael Apple
& Rowena Gaunt

metro

First published in Great Britain in 1998
by Metro Books (an imprint of Metro Publishing Limited),
19 Gerrard Street, London W1V 7LA

British Library Cataloguing in Publication Data. A CIP record
of this book is available on request from the British Library.

Cover design by David Farrow

ISBN 1 900512 39 4

10 9 8 7 6 5 4 3 2 1

Typeset by Wakewing, High Wycombe
Printed in Great Britain by CPD Group, Wales

Acknowledgements

With thanks to our agent, Teresa Chris, and to Metro Publishing, especially for the perceptive input from Mary Remnant.

Of the many reference books we consulted particularly important were *The Oxford Textbook of Medicine* (OUP, 1996), *Clinical Medicine* (Kumar and Clark, Bailiere Tindall, 1994), and *The Hamlyn Encyclopaedia of Complementary Health* (Hamlyn, 1966). However, the opinions stated in this book are entirely our own, as is the responsibility for any errors.

For JP, Marilyn, Zoë and Daniel

Contents

Introduction

MODERN MAN – CAN HE HAVE IT ALL?

Whatever your age, marital status or occupation, your health can affect all aspects of your life. Looking briefly at three very different modern men helps to explain this.

Tom is in his late twenties. His work involves constant pressures to achieve, in an atmosphere of goals, targets, and fierce competition. But that same pressure gives Tom a thrill; he knows he can deliver to deadlines, he knows he has the edge over his colleagues, he can think on his feet and make his own luck. Life is frantic. But Tom is also self-aware enough to know that he must lay the basis for a healthy life, even if he can scarcely find time to brush his teeth. This book shows how you can channel vitality towards healthy goals.

James is more established and is a family man. At work he rules the roost, confident in his know-how and contacts. But at home his baby is a money-pit, and his older children drop hints about loss of face if they cannot have designer gear. He gets out of breath when playing with them and wonders if this is serious. His partner is pursuing her own career, and he suspects she is rather better at hers than he is at his own. James has reached a stage in his life when he has to confront the limits of his physical and mental abilities.

Later, in bed, James turns uncertainly to his partner, a jumble of thoughts in his head: 'She's had a hard day too; last time she seemed bored, and after all that wine it never quite seems to work! Maybe I'm too old anyway.' He turns back and mutters good night thinking to himself 'Here comes old age'. It does not have to be this way.

Then there are Bob and Carol. Bob has made it. Their life is affluent; holidays are good, they eat well, there is a new car on the drive. They meet their friends in restaurants or at the theatre. The pace is less frenetic and Bob gets an opportunity to review his life with leisure. What should he do about that tightening in his chest, the surge of acid that reminds him how much he's eaten and his aching muscles when he plays golf? When should he worry about his health? Not for the first time, he answers himself, 'Tomorrow. That's when I'll deal with my health.'

Perhaps you recognize yourself in one of these scenarios, though not all the details fit – you may be single, childless, gay or self-employed. Even so, chances are you are not immune to wounded male pride, worry about work, money or the external stresses of life. If you want to do something about it, and want to regain control of your life, this book will show you how.

In our advice on how to improve your health, we have taken a holistic approach to all aspects of your well-being – not just your body, or your image, or your sex-appeal or your spirit, but all these aspects of your personality, and others too. When you've finished reading, you'll be able to face life with confidence, self-esteem, and a positive attitude.

WHY NOW?

For too long men's health has been neglected. Everyone vaguely knows that men get heart disease, prostate trouble and dodgy hips, but that's life isn't it? And as for those psychological things like nerves and depression, what's wrong that can't be cured by a drink with your mates and a few cigarettes?

Some men think that while women get menopausal and droopy as they age, their own sex somehow matures and solidifies, a reflection of a good life and honest worry. And so when a friend pops his clogs aged fifty, a man can tell himself that the other bloke had fought the good fight and kept up his life insurance. He himself might have to get up a few times a night to have a pee, but he can congratulate himself that he at least has made it to retirement.

ON NOT MAKING A FUSS

This same attitude of inevitability extends to worrying symptoms. Flecks of blood in the motions are only piles. A persistent cough must be due to pollution. Trembling hands are surely just from too much coffee. Men call this being realistic.

OF MEN AND MEDICS

What discourages men from going to the doctor? One problem is that it takes an unusual effort. Whereas for most women medical attention is almost inevitable – they see the doctor about their periods, contraception, pregnancy and the menopause, as well as taking their children for check-ups – men have a gloomy feeling that if they go to the doctor he or she will only find something wrong. It is the 'my car goes 50,000 miles between oil changes and runs perfectly' school of health care.

Doctors do realize that men are apt to make light of their symptoms. They know that men have a different style of consultation, tending to say what they think is wrong (the diagnosis) rather than relating how they feel (the symptoms) and leaving it to the doctor to interpret for them. A typical conversation might go:

'I've got indigestion, Doc, that white medicine helped me last time.'
'What type of discomfort are you getting and where?'
'It's indigestion pain, Doc, and I get it here.' (pointing to the heart)
'Does eating bring it on, or anything else?'
'Sometimes. Oh yes, and if I'm in a hurry or going up a hill.'
'It sounds like I'd better check your heart.'
'Ah come on Doc, you're a busy person, give me the right medicine and I'll go'
'Just take your shirt off, please.'

As men become more health aware, their reluctance to confront problems is changing; this is something that doctors welcome. It is now common for men to go to their GP specifically for a blood-pressure test, a or general check-over.

Well-man clinics are widely available and remove the element of making a fuss from going to the doctor. They also make an appointment more like a business meeting: a booked time, an agenda, exchange of information and agreeing a strategy for the next few months.

Just like a business meeting, to be successful a medical consultation involves:

- good disclosure of information, i.e. honest answers to questions;
- negotiation ('Tell you what Doc, I'll drop to ten cigarettes a day to start with');

- subtle ploys ('If you could lose weight you might not need those tablets that affect your sex life');
- ultimatums ('the last patient who said they'd think about tests died three weeks later');
- agreement about conclusions and a decision about the next date for a meeting;
- expression of mutual admiration and handshakes.

WHY THINGS ARE CHANGING

Men are now increasingly looking at the quality of their lives, and not just at mere survival. Ours is an affluent society where despite the pressures, life is better for many people than it ever was in the past. It follows that both men and women want to take full advantage of life and of the extended retirements that they can expect.

IMAGE

Being able to maximize the pleasures of life is a personal gain. A more public benefit is from being seen to be healthy – a valuable asset in a stressful, competitive and image-obsessed society.

You may not be concerned about someone's health as long as he does the job; but in reality wouldn't you rather put your trust in an insurance agent who looks slim and fit, or a pilot who looks alert but relaxed or a surgeon with steady hands? And in the middle of an important business deal, could you completely put out of your mind the knowledge that a colleague's concentration is currently affected by a relationship problem?

With these sorts of pressures, it is not surprising that men increasingly want to be seen as healthy and stable, and to project positive images through their lifestyle, dress, posture and speech. Health can mean wealth.

It is an outdated belief that early death from male diseases is inevitable; men are ever more concerned to preserve health and vigour. Widely publicized evidence shows that men who exercise regularly and eat a healthy diet live longer and better. Taking care of your health is respectable, and no longer a fringe activity for a few committed enthusiasts.

Research is increasingly confirming the value of early intervention in high blood pressure, prostate diseases, diabetes etc.

The medicines for these, and many other conditions, have become more convenient to take and have fewer side-effects than in the past.

Advances are also being made in treating diseases where until recently no treatment was possible. Many of these are predominately male diseases, such as heart attacks or coronary artery disease, the handling of which has been transformed in the last ten years.

Good health, physical and mental, is a bulwark against the stresses of our society. In the first century AD Juvenal advised that you should pray to have a healthy mind in a healthy body. It is unfortunate that such an ancient truth has so frequently been ignored.

Women have had a key role in changing male attitudes to well-being. They have always been more health aware than men, an awareness forced on them by responsibilities for themselves and for the babies they nurture, and they want to share health benefits with their male partners.

Though perfect health is rarely attainable and ageing cannot be halted, much can be done to make male maturity pleasant and enjoyable.

Quiz

Although men tend to be far more ignorant than women about their health – in body, mind and spirit – this book can help you change that. But in order to change, you need to know where you start, so answer the questions below to find out if there are any gaps in your knowledge.

BODY

1   What is the risk you will die of testicular cancer?
a) 1 in 300
b) 1 in 450
c) 1 in 750

2   What is the number one killer for all men?
a) Heart disease
b) Lung cancer
c) Alzheimer's disease

3   What is the ideal number of calories the average male should consume each day?
a) 2,550
b) 3,550
c) 4,550

4   Where is your prostate gland?
a) At the base of your throat, just under your Adam's apple
b) In the middle of the underside of your brain
c) Immediately under your bladder

5   What is chlamydia?
a) A viral infection of the lungs, which can lead to chronic bronchitis
b) A bacterial infection of the eyes which can lead to glaucoma
c) A bacterial sexually transmitted disease (STD) which is usually symptomless, but can lead to sub-fertility in women

6   Under most circumstances, is it usually best for the health of new babies if they are:
a) Breast fed
b) Bottle fed
c) Offered mixed feeding – breast and bottle

MIND

7 Men are more likely to suffer depression than women.
a) True
b) False
c) Men and women are equally likely to suffer depression

8 Men's adrenaline levels rise when they are under stress.
a) Always true
b) Sometimes true, depending on the circumstances
c) Adrenaline is a female hormone

9 Which of the following most often causes men anxiety?
a) Work
b) Emotional aspects of relationships
c) Sexual performance

10 Suicide is the leading cause of death in men aged sixteen to twenty-four.
a) True
b) False

11 Your brain has a vast over-capacity, so it doesn't matter if you kill a few of its cells through drinking.
a) True
b) False

SPIRIT

12 What is aurasoma?
a) The unique energy field that each of us possesses
b) A complementary therapy combining aromatherapy and colour therapy
c) A yoga position

13 What is the best way of getting out of trouble with women?
a) Lying
b) Pleading
c) Crying

14 The purpose of sex is:
a) Recreation
b) Procreation
c) A way to express love, respect and honour for your partner

15 Which of the following things about men most infuriate women?
a) Men don't communicate their feelings
b) Men are frightened of commitment
c) Men are unfaithful

ANSWERS AND ANALYSIS

BODY

1 The answer is 1 in 450. The risk of developing testicular cancer has doubled in the last twenty years. Every man should check his testicles at least once a month. For advice on how to do so, and what to look for, see page 54.

2 Heart disease. This kills 50 per cent of men. For advice on reducing your risk, see page 51. Lung cancer kills over 20,000 men a year, and Alzheimer's disease affects one in five men over eighty.

3 2,550 calories. An inactive twenty-five year old weighing 9 stone needs only 2,220, while an active thirty-five year old weighing 12 stone can tuck away 3,940. For advice on diet, see pages 13 and 24.

4 Your prostate is immediately under your bladder. Prostate cancer affects many men over seventy, and benign enlargement is common. See page 53 for more details. The gland under your Adam's Apple is the thyroid, which secretes hormones regulating metabolism, and the one in your brain is the pituitary, which controls your entire hormonal system.

5 Chlamydia is an STD which is symptomless in men, but which can have terrible consequences for women, who may become infertile as a result of infection. See page 96, and if there is any chance you might be infected, seek a medical opinion as a matter of urgency.

6 No woman should ever feel bullied into adopting one or other policy, but breast is usually best, for all sorts of reasons. For discussion of the emotional upheaval of becoming a father, and supporting your partner at this time, see page 114.

MIND

7 Women are more likely to seek help for depression than men. However, once postnatal depression is excluded, it is likely that the sexes experience depression in equal numbers – men just don't like to admit it. For advice on depression see page 150.

8 In both men and women, adrenaline levels always rise under stress. For stress-busting strategies, see page 140.

9 About 25 per cent of men suffer severe anxiety and all three of these are significant triggers, but emotional aspects of relationships are the factors most frequently mentioned in surveys. See page 145 for advice on coping with anxiety and panic attacks.

10 Sadly, it's true. Young men are at significantly greater risk of suicide than young women. See page 57 for further details.

11 This widely held belief is false. See page 33 for strategies for reducing your alcohol intake.

SPIRIT

12 Aurasoma is a complementary therapy. Men can benefit hugely from complementary therapies, and advice and information is included throughout this book. Your unique energy field is your aura.

13 This is a trick question – it depends on the woman. Any of these could work, any could result in a clip around the ear. See Part Two for a trip through the minefield of male/female relationships.

14 This is another trick question. The biological purpose of sex is procreation, but for most of us most of the time, sex is a combination of all three – sometimes one element predominates, sometimes another. Again, see Part Two.

15 Women are driven to distraction by men who won't communicate feelings. They are irritated by men's fears of commitment, and are infuriated by infidelity. See Part Two.

HOW MANY DID YOU GET RIGHT?

1–5? It's surprising you're not dead! You really need to study this book, and to ask yourself some searching questions about how well you understand yourself and women.

6–10? You have a typically average understanding of male health, in its broadest interpretation. Complete all our programmes for change and you'll find new avenues for growth and self-development opening out before you.

11–15? What a paragon! You are already aware of your health-related needs and can see all the benefits of taking a holistic approach to your well-being.

WHO ARE THE HEALTH HEROES?

Men who read this book have the chance of becoming health heroes – heroes in their own eyes and in the eyes of those who love them and depend on them.

What do you think makes a hero? Is he a demigod? A man of superhuman qualities? A man admired for great deeds and noble attributes? Is he the strong, silent type, or would he be prepared to cry on occasion?

You cannot become a hero before you know what you mean by a hero. This book cannot tell you what it would mean for you to become one – only you can decide that, and there are no easy answers.

However, whatever else it means, becoming a hero means being willing to change. It means being prepared to put aside old ways of thinking. It means opening up to ever-expanding networks of possibilities.

From ancient Greece to the modern day, heroes have been quick-thinking, adaptable, innovative – the men prepared to exploit altered circumstances and new situations, to thrive when all about them have been floundering.

What's this got to do with health? As we've already seen, for their own good, and for the good of those they love, men's attitudes to their own well-being need to change. To grasp this, and to be prepared to do something about it, requires the basic heroic qualities of vision and versatility.

Have you got these qualities? In this book, we will provide all the basic information needed to spur you into new ways of thinking. We'll also provide four programmes for change. If you are prepared to follow them, to throw out treasured prejudices, misconceptions and preconceived ideas, then you really will have become a health hero: a man who can be proud of himself, and of whom others can be proud. See page 195 for the benefits of becoming a health hero.

PART ONE
physical HeaLTH

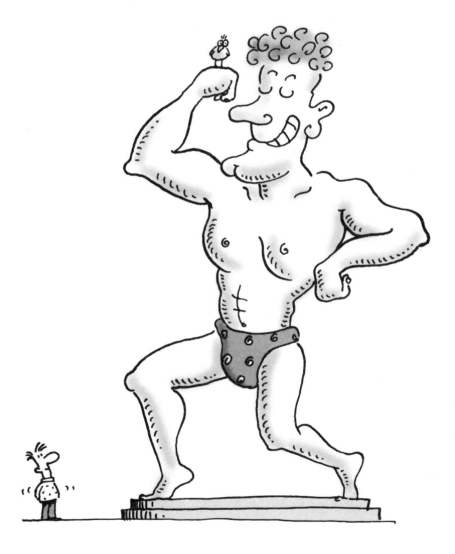

Diet and Nutrition

A good diet is one in which the food you eat contains all the nutrients needed by the body to promote physical, mental, emotional and spiritual health. A bad diet can contribute to obesity, heart disease, cancer, digestive disorders, mood-swings, irritability, and insomnia – to name just a few problems.

Ideally, your diet should contain a balanced mix of foods from the three food groups:

- Protein – from meat, dairy produce, eggs, fish, poultry, pulses, nuts and seeds. Protein should make up about 15 per cent of your diet. Try to have two servings a day of non-dairy produce, and one serving of a dairy product.
- Carbohydrate – from bread, pasta, rice, potatoes, pulses, nuts and seeds, fruit, vegetables and salads. Carbohydrates should make up about 60 per cent of your diet. Try to have five servings a day of fruit, vegetables or salads, and four servings of carbohydrates from other sources.
- Fat – found in most foods, except fruit, vegetables, and salad (although avocados contain fat). Too much of the wrong sort of fat is bad for you. Try not to add fat to your food, and remove excess fat before you cook meat. Take the skin off poultry. Avoid fats which are solid at room temperature, e.g. lard and butter. Fats which are liquid at room temperature, i.e. all vegetable oils, are far preferable. This is because fats which are liquid at room temperature do not contain the chemicals which can ultimately lead to clogging of the arteries, whereas fats which are solid at room temperature do. Fat should make up a maximum of 30 per cent of your diet.

VITAMINS AND MINERALS

Vitamins and minerals are vital for health because both clinical and sub-clinical deficiencies can play havoc with your body. A clinical deficiency results in a condition (e.g. pernicious anaemia caused by a lack of vitamin B12) which would be recognized and treated by orthodox medicine. A sub-clinical deficiency leads to a range of niggling health problems which undermine well-being but are not normally treated by orthodox medical practitioners. If you eat a cross-section of foods from the three groups, you should, in theory, get all the vitamins and minerals you need. However, even fresh wholefoods can be less nutritious than you might think. Nutrients can be leached from our food in a variety of hidden ways, and chemicals are often added. For example:

- soil and water are often contaminated with industrial or agricultural contaminants;
- intensive farming methods make heavy use of pesticides, antibiotics and growth promoters;
- long storage or transit times can alter the structure of food, without rendering it inedible;
- pre-prepared or processed foods are likely to have added colorants, preservatives, flavourings, emulsifiers and polyphosphates;
- freezing and canning can remove vitamins and minerals.

In addition, alcohol, drugs, tobacco, stress and environmental pollution can deplete the body of essential nutrients. For all these reasons, you might want to supplement your diet with extra vitamins and minerals, available from pharmacies, health food stores and supermarkets. Also, try to buy organic. This might be difficult, and certainly more expensive than buying mass-produced food, but what you eat will be free of organophosphates, which can damage the nervous system.

COMMON VITAMINS	Found in	Good for
Vitamin A	liver, carrots, green vegetables	skin and, especially, eyes
B group vitamins	Marmite, bread, breakfast cereal, dairy products, vegetables	nervous system and circulation
Vitamin C	citrus fruits, potatoes, green vegetables	immune system, absorption of iron and folic acid

Vitamin D	oily fish, salmon, dairy products	bones and teeth
Vitamin E	nuts, seeds, vegetable oils	fat metabolism, and nervous system

Vitamins A, C and E are anti-oxidant, which means they can help the body break down otherwise harmful chemicals, thus possibly protecting us from cancer.

Warning! Some vitamins can be toxic, if taken in excess – e.g. vitamin A. If in doubt, consult a pharmacist, doctor or nutritional therapist.

COMMON MINERALS	*Found in*	*Good for*
Calcium	milk, cheese, watercress	bones, teeth, blood clotting
Chromium	egg yolk, wheatgerm, chicken	sugar metabolism, and blood pressure
Copper	most foods	healthy connective tissues
Iron	liver, dried fruit, meat green vegetables	blood, circulatory and immune systems
Magnesium	nuts, chicken, cheese	muscles and nervous system
Potassium	raisins, potatoes, fruit and vegetables	nerve transmission, acid/alkaline balance in our bodies
Selenium	kidney, liver, red meat	heart and liver
Zinc	cheese, wholemeal bread, eggs	reproductive system, hair and nails

Selenium is anti-oxidant, which means it can help the body break down otherwise harmful chemicals, thus possibly protecting us from cancer.

Warning! Some minerals can be toxic, if taken in excess. If in doubt, consult a pharmacist, doctor or nutritional therapist.

DIETARY FIBRE

Fibre swells the bulk of the food residue in the intestine, and helps to soften it by increasing the amount of water retained. It is vital to the health of the digestive system, and many ailments can result if we do not get enough, e.g. irritable bowel syndrome, constipation and haemorrhoids (piles). Western diets tend to be low in fibre, because we eat so much processed and refined food. Even in the most hectic of lives, there are easy ways to boost fibre:

- Start the day with a bowl of high-fibre cereal. If you eat breakfast at work, take in a box of cereal at the beginning of the week, rather than buying a croissant or doughnut from the local coffee shop each morning.
- Eat wholemeal bread. If you buy sandwiches for lunch, choose brown bread. (Wholemeal pasta and brown rice are good for you too, though to begin with they may be an acquired taste.)
- Change your snacking habits. Fruit or nuts are healthier snacks than chocolate or biscuits.

High-fibre foods are nutritious without containing concentrated calories, fat, sugar or salt. They tend to be filling without being fattening. Some types of fibre – that found in vegetables, fruit, pulses and oats – can help reduce blood cholesterol levels. Cholesterol is a type of fat which is implicated in clogging of the arteries with atheroma (a greasy material), especially the arteries around the heart. However, cholesterol is not an entirely undesirable molecule as we need it to keep our nervous systems healthy.

You should try to eat at least 30g of fibre per day, from a selection of foods. The table below will help you calculate what you should eat. It includes some commonly eaten higher fibre foods. As well as supplying fibre, many of these also supply carbohydrate (starch) and other essentials of a balanced diet.

FOOD	Fibre in grammes per ounce	Fibre in grammes per typical helping
White bread	0.8	0.8 per slice
Wholemeal bread	2.4	2.4 per slice
Cornflakes	0.9	1.0
Muesli	2.0	4.0
Bran cereals	4–8.0	8–16.0
Rice (white, boiled)	0.2	0.6
Rice (brown, boiled)	0.4	1.2
Mushrooms	0.7	1.4
Cabbage	1.0	3–4.0
Broccoli	1.1	2–3.0
Carrots	0.9	2–3.0
Pasta (white)	0.2	1.0
Pasta (brown)	0.9	4–5.0
Potatoes (boiled)	0.3	2–3.0
Potatoes (jacket)	0.7	5–8.0
Chips	0.6	3–6.0
Crisps	3.2	3.2
	(NB: these are high in calories)	
Baked beans	2.0	8.0
Peas	2.0	4.0
Bananas	1.0	4.0
	(NB: most soft fruit is low in fibre)	
Prunes (dried)	3.8	8–12.0
Peanuts	2.3	4–6
	(NB: these are also high in calories)	

WATER AND ALCOHOL

You are probably not drinking enough water, which is an important part of diet – it helps flush toxins out of the body. Ideally, you should drink at least three litres of water a day to maintain health – if you work in an office, keep a bottle on your desk.

Try to cut down on alcohol – among other things, it is very calorific and will encourage weight gain. When you have a drink, make sure you also have something to eat.

SALT AND SUGAR

Many processed foods contain salt, which contributes to high blood pressure. Try to avoid such foods; do not sprinkle salt on your vegetables, and stop buying crisps.

Refined white sugar is bad for you; it rots your teeth, sends your blood-sugar levels haywire, making you subject to mood swings, and provides you with a shot of empty calories which go straight to your waistline. If you have a sweet tooth, try to eat fruit rather than sweets, biscuits or cakes.

CAN'T COOK, WON'T COOK!

Even if you never have time to shop, do not know how to cook, and eat out or buy take-aways all the time, there are still simple steps you can take to improve your diet:

- Think about the choices you are making. Fried egg and chips are nice, but scrambled eggs and a baked potato are better for you. Even the very worst work canteen is likely to offer this sort of choice – and certainly the better restaurants.
- Check the labels on ready-made products – particularly for the fat content. As a rough guide, try to choose dishes containing less than 5g of fat per serving.
- At lunch, don't buy a burger, go for a salad box.
- When eating out, choose plain grilled meat, fish or poultry, rather than something more fancy. Avoid gravies and sauces made with cream or butter.
- Don't eat fried, deep fried or sautéed food.
- If you live off toast, make sure it's wholemeal, and spread it with yeast extract or peanut butter, not jam. Beans on toast provides all the nutrients you need. Pilchards on toast is quick, easy and nutritious – oily fish, like mackerel and pilchards, contain oils which can help prevent the onset of heart disease.
- If you are eating a pizza, order a thin and crispy base, not deep crust, and choose vegetable toppings – pepperoni is not a healthy option.
- If you are having an Indian, pass on the poppadoms and pickles; try to stick to dry cooked meats and choose plenty of vegetables.
- If you like Chinese food, try to choose vegetable dishes, and go for rice, not noodles.

- Think about when you eat as well as what you eat – it's better to have small, regular meals, than a daily blow-out.
- Don't skip breakfast – here are three reasons why. You will be hungry all morning and tempted to snack on unhealthy instant sources of energy such as chocolate biscuits. You might experience low blood sugar, with light-headedness and irritability. This might lead you not to think as clearly, concentrate as well or act as decisively as if you eat something first thing. You will be tempted to eat a much larger lunch than is wise, which will make you sleepy in the afternoon.
- Think about taking nutritional supplements, not just the vitamins mentioned above but also those in the table below. All should be available from your local health store.

WORST-CASE MEALS
Breakfast: Danish pastry and a cappuccino at your desk, or bacon, egg and sausage.
Lunch: burger and fries and a Mars Bar, or meat pie and chips.
Dinner: curry, rice, poppadoms and pickles, washed down with six pints of lager, or a take-away deep-crust pepperoni pizza.

HEALTHY ALTERNATIVES
Breakfast: a bowl of cereal at your desk with orange juice, or poached eggs on toast.
Lunch: salad box and a piece of fruit, or chicken salad sandwiches without mayonnaise and with a piece of fruit.
Dinner: Indian – choose a dry dish e.g. chicken sashlick or tikka, or Italian – go for pasta with a simple vegetable sauce.

Dietary supplement	Good for
Evening Primrose Oil	skin; also to regulate cholesterol and blood pressure
Fish oils	heart; and to promote mental agility
Garlic	lungs and the immune system
Ginseng	mental health and stamina
Lecithin	heart and circulatory system
Royal Jelly	stamina and energy levels

NUTRITIONAL THERAPY

Nutritional therapy uses diet and vitamin and mineral supplementation to balance the body and prevent illness. There are three basic diagnoses: food intolerance, nutritional deficiency and toxic overload. See Appendix for more details.

Beer bellies and spare tyres

EATING FOR HEALTH

If someone makes fun of your sagging stomach will you ever do something about it? This section gives you some reasons to think about tackling being overweight, the principles of dieting and how to go about changing your eating habits.

Why bother?

During the last hundred years, heart disease has moved from being a rarity to being one of the two major causes of death (the other is cancer). As an unfortunate fact, men are most affected by heart trouble. The experts are still in dispute about why this is the case, but diet seems to be a major explanation. Several studies have traced how heart disease increases in immigrants as they move away from a more basic Third World diet to a Western diet, with increased amounts of fat. The Western diet also lacks the green leafy vegetables containing vitamin E. This anti-oxidant mops up free radicals. These are naturally occurring biochemicals released during metabolism. Their role in heart disease is still poorly understood but they appear to be important in causing heart trouble.

Apart from not eating well, we tend to eat too much. There is an epidemic of obesity in the West. Obesity not only offers the prospect of heart attacks but also leads to diabetes and the physical side-effects of obesity such as arthritis, tiredness, and skin rashes.

Are you alarmed yet? Consider in addition that the foods we eat tend to contain less fibre, which it seems likely predisposes to bowel disorders such as diverticulitis and possibly even bowel cancer.

Convenience food.

This may taste nice but is not always good for you. Besides a high fat content, pizzas, fry-ups and take-away snacks contain salt which leads to high blood pressure and possibly heart disease, and sugar which predisposes to tooth decay, obesity and diabetes.

Where the fat goes

Men tend to put on excess weight around the waist – as opposed to the hips, which is more where women accumulate fat. This is important because fat around the waist corresponds to fat accumulating within the abdominal cavity and it is this centrally held fat which appears most important in generating the health problems caused by obesity.

Beer bellies

For reasons not understood, a high alcohol intake tends to produce fat laid down within the abdomen, rather than the buttocks. This is the origin of the familiar beer belly and is a risk marker for heart disease for the reasons given earlier.

Big is not necessarily fat

A big and heavy man may be mainly muscle, whereas a much lighter man may be carrying far more by way of fat. This can easily be recognized by doctors. They use an index called body mass index (BMI), which relates height to weight. The formula is your weight in kilograms divided by your height in metres squared. An index above 30 means obesity serious enough to affect health.

HOW TO ADJUST YOUR DIET

Diets to lose weight

To lose weight you must either reduce your food intake or increase activity – and preferably both. As a first step, you need to calculate how much energy you require, measured in calories; you will have to restrict calories to lose weight. Many people originally gain excess calories (and therefore excess weight) from carbohydrate. This is found in starchy foods like sugar, cakes, biscuits, beer and especially in snacks and convenience foods.

As a guide, men aged between nineteen and sixty doing a sedentary job require 2,550 calories a day; someone in a physically demanding job may need up to 4,000 calories a day. In these situations, as long as intake matches output, overall weight remains steady, with no tendency to accumulate fat.

A balanced diet

Knowing your calorie requirements, you can calculate what your diet should contain in order either to lose weight or to maintain a healthy weight. You get energy from carbohydrates, fat and protein. Other guidance is given elsewhere in this chapter and in the tables.

Choosing a diet

Check your desirable weight in the table below, or speak to your doctor or a dietitian.

HEIGHT	Acceptable range	Obese
160cm/5ft 3in	52–65kg/8st 3lb–10st 3lb	78kg/12st 5lb
162cm/5ft 4in	53–66kg/8st 5lb–10st 5lb	79kg/12st 6lb
166cm/5ft 5in	55–69kg/8st 11lb–10st 12lb	83kg/13st
170cm/5ft 7in	58–73kg/9st 2lb–11 7lb	88kg/13st 12lb
176cm/5ft 9in	62–77kg/9st 10lb–12st 2lb	92kg/14st 7lb
180cm/5ft 10½in	65–80kg/10st 3lb–12st 8lb	96kg/15st 2lb
184cm/6ft	67–84kg/10st 8lb–13st 3lb	101kg/16st
190cm/6ft 2in	73–90kg/11st 7lb–14st 2lb	108kg/17st
192cm/6ft 4in	75–93kg/11 st 11lb–14st 10lb	112kg/17½st

Do not imagine that you can lose excess weight in one great effort. During a crash diet, all you will lose is fluid, which will re-accumulate rapidly. Instead, aim to lose a pound or so a week. Does this sound too wimpish for you? Over three months you will lose a stone – and four stone over a year. This is major-league weight loss. Remember, it took you years to acquire that gently rounded and sagging look, so you won't be able to shed it rapidly.

Save me from the lettuce leaf

Fear not; to diet successfully you need not smuggle in pots of low-fat yogurt and leafy salads – unless you want to. In fact you could probably eat much of what you eat now, just eat less of it and ensure proper quantities of vital extras such as vitamins and minerals.

Diets to stay healthy

Carbohydrate sources are pasta, rice, potatoes, bread. These should increase. The quantity should supply the calories you have calculated you need, less that supplied by fat in your diet.

FIBRE

This comes from vegetable products, high-fibre breads, and fruit. You should have 30g a day.

FAT

Your total fat intake should be limited to 77–87g a day, which will provide you with 31–34 per cent of energy (calories). Choose fat sources containing low cholesterol and that are high in polyunsaturated fats as in fish, nuts, sunflower and soya oils, and soft margarines. Avoid animal fats, dripping, bacon, sausages, hard margarines, pastries and cakes.

FOOD GROUPS

Meat, fish, eggs, pulses, nuts

Milk, cheese and dairy products

Fruit and vegetables

Cereals (including bread, pasta, rice)

SALT

Salt is ubiquitous in crisps, snacks, and processed foods. The World Health Organization recommends no more than 5g a day. Do not automatically pour salt over your food. Taste it before you reach for the salt cellar. Each week, make yourself eat food with a little less salt in it.

VITAMINS

These chemicals are needed in minute amounts for essential body functions but the body is unable to make vitamins for itself. Vitamin deficiency is only likely if you are deliberately neglecting yourself – especially if you are alcoholic, or relying on alcohol to supply you with carbohydrates.

MINERALS

The body requires many simple elements such as iron, zinc, copper, selenium, calcium, sodium and potassium. You may not get these if you follow an extreme diet – for instance, if you restrict yourself to one type of food.

HEALTHY EATING

On a daily basis:

- Eat something from each food group.
- Select reduced fat milk and dairy products.
- Select lean (fat-trimmed) meat or else pulses, fish, dried beans, lentils.
- Eat some bread and cereal – wholegrain if possible.
- Eat three vegetables and two fruits (fresh, frozen or canned, it makes no difference). Juice and salads count towards this.
- Choose foods low in salt, sugar and saturated fat – food labels help in this selection.

Losing weight – the principles

- Work out a target weight.
- List your food intake. You should particularly remember to note 'empty' calories from alcohol, sweet drinks, snacks, crisps, sweets and chocolate.
- Settle on a balanced diet with variety, as you are more likely to persevere with this.
- Put your food on smaller plates and eat more slowly (simple but effective). For similar reasons, do not eat while watching TV, a sports match or anything else which takes your mind off how much you are shovelling in.
- Can you persuade a friend to diet with you? – someone who gets as out of breath as you do and so has similar reasons to persevere.
- Aim to lose a steady half to one pound a week.
- As well as dieting, increase your exercise – three half-hour walks a week is a good start.
- Think of a reward for your effort – though the approval of your girlfriend and workmates may be enough.
- Be prepared to be teased by people; just remember, you may yet be visiting them after they have developed diabetes or had a heart attack.

Always take professional advice before embarking on a major diet or exercise regime.

Sport, exercise and training

What would men do if they did not have sport and exercise? A large proportion of their time is spent participating in, watching or shouting at sport. This must meet some deep needs. The possibilities include:

- The sheer pleasure from honing your body to peak perfection and using it to its fullest capabilities.
- Innate male competitiveness to succeed – physical exertion is an arena for competition.
- Innate male behaviour, pre-wired in the brain, hormone-driven and an end in itself.
- A biologically pre-set behaviour, designed to enable women to select their mate, attracted by the man who is successful, biggest, fastest etc.
- As a career, offering an attractive future for a determined, naturally talented man.
- Companionship, shared aspirations, joint pleasure and male bonding.
- Any and all of these.

SPORT FOR HEALTH

In addition to all the above, active participation in sport can help men with an innate problem. This is that the male hormones that help you to enjoy sport also increase your risk of heart disease. Men are forty times at more risk of heart trouble than women up to the menopause (after that, the risks gradually get the same). Exercise reduces the risk (but you should also quit smoking and have the other health checks specified on page 45 onwards).

THE BENEFITS OF EXERCISE

Apart from feeling fitter and generally more healthy, you will get:

- a stronger heart;
- reduced risks of heart attack and strokes;
- more efficient muscles;
- improved general blood flow;
- lower blood cholesterol;
- a sense of well-being;
- stamina.

HOW FIT CAN I GET?

It is far easier to move from unfit to fitter than it is to move from very fit to super fit. Significantly increased exercise ability can be seen after just two to three weeks and major effects on stamina after three to four months. Of course, we all have genetically determined limits on how fit we can get, so there may be limits which are always beyond you.

What do you have to do to achieve fitness? Don't panic. Even three brisk twenty-minute walks (at greater than 4 mph) a week will provide a substantial benefit to your heart and general well-being. Here is some more information about sport and exercise.

THE RAW INGREDIENTS

You start with what you have – your natural shape, musculature and flexibility. These biological factors determine what you will be best at – heavily muscled men make good sprinters, rowers, rugby players; slim ones long-distance runners. Whatever the starting position, you can always improve on it by training. Training enhances your innate energy system, by gradually increasing the demands made of it. Training will improve the heart, the muscles, and the blood vessels. The benefits will become clear after just a few weeks of training, when you will already notice improved stamina and less breathlessness. And this is a benefit whatever your level of fitness at the outset.

HOW MUSCLES WORK

There are several different types of muscle. The ones you use when exercising are made up of innumerable fibres arranged in sequence and ending in a tendon that attaches the muscle to a bone. Movement is produced by contraction of muscle fibres, which causes the bone to move. The process of contraction is still not fully understood but appears to involve molecules within the muscle fibres sliding over each other, using energy to do so. This energy comes from glycogen (stored sugar). If the body runs out of sugar it can get energy by breaking down fat or protein for a while.

AEROBIC AND ANAEROBIC ENERGY

To burn sugar as fuel requires oxygen, which we get by breathing and is transmitted to muscle through the blood supply. As long as there is plenty of oxygen around, the body produces energy in an efficient process called aerobic energy production. Should oxygen be scarce, perhaps when sprinting or during a sudden burst of physical activity, there may not be enough oxygen to produce energy through these usual aerobic channels. The body can turn automatically to energy pathways which are anaerobic (literally, without air). These biochemical pathways supply the energy but at a cost of an accumulation of waste products, especially lactic acid; these can only be got rid of once there is plenty of oxygen available. This is called an oxygen debt and is one reason for the feeling of exhaustion and the heavy deep breathing after strenuous exercise. Whenever you exercise, to start with your energy comes from anaerobic pathways; the aerobic pathways take a few minutes to kick in.

TRAINING

During training you are pushing your body to perform harder, longer and more frequently. The body has automatic mechanisms which respond to these demands by gradually increasing the size of muscle fibres and making them more efficient at using energy. The blood supply to muscles improves, and the heart (which is also muscle) responds by growing and pumping more efficiently. Your lung capacity increases so providing more oxygen. A fully trained individual can deliver more blood more quickly for longer to the body, while his muscles can produce more power for extended periods of time.

MEASURING TRAINING

The maximum heart rate is a good indication of training for most purposes, though specialized fitness laboratories can measure the actual energy being expended along with oxygen consumption. A training programme will start by determining what your maximum heart rate is after steady exertion – running, jogging etc. A training programme will set you targets that raise your heart rate to 60–85 per cent of that maximum for at least twenty minutes at time. Those sessions should be repeated two or three times a week. Exercises to achieve this are jogging, running, stepping, cycling – in fact typical exercises that you will find equipment for in a gym.

Such exercise is beneficial to the whole body, improving heart, lungs, blood flow and muscles generally. If in addition you want to strengthen individual muscles, then you must turn to more specific equipment – perhaps to stretch your thigh muscles, your pectorals and your shoulder muscles.

WARMING UP AND COOLING DOWN

You cannot expect your muscles to perform at maximum efficiency instantly, any more than you can race your car from a cold start. You have to let them warm up, during which time the blood flow increases and the aerobic pathways get into action. A typical warm-up session takes just ten minutes, during which you should be stretching those muscles and tendons which your exercise or sport requires, and putting enough effort into it to make yourself break out in a mild sweat. During a warm-up the balance of blood flow to muscle increases from a resting 15–20 per cent of total heart output to a remarkable 70 per cent, and the power your muscles can deliver increases correspondingly. In this way your body is at peak performance when you begin your sport and the chances of injuring muscles or tendons are reduced.

After exercise

After a demanding game it is as important to cool down in a planned way. This is because your body is bound to have built up some waste lactic acid and therefore has an oxygen debt to pay off. Were you to stop suddenly, the waste products would tend to cause cramp, aching muscles and overwhelming fatigue as well as leaving you gasping for an inelegant ten minutes. It's better, therefore, to finish off with a gentle jog or brisk walking to keep blood flowing vigorously through your muscles, flushing away waste products. So much the better if you can make this your victory jog round the arena!

ATTITUDE

Psychology is important in achieving peak competitive performance; top athletes learn to think themselves into success in order to gain that tiny additional edge critical to maximum performance. Hyping yourself up for a five-a-side football match on your local pitch is not in the same league. Nevertheless all competition benefits from some simple mental preparation.

- Understand the game and your role in it – are you a supporting player, or are you expected to make your own luck and to seize every opportunity?
- Know the rules – you may not follow them but at least breaking them then becomes a matter of calculation rather than mishap.
- Respect your opponents – if you think you are good, the people you are playing against are likely to be good too; underestimating them will lead to surprise at their abilities, then disappointment that will take the edge off your performance.
- Think back to your previous best performances; savour the excitement, the buzz, the applause.
- Expect to win but not necessarily from the start; know that you have reserves of psychological and physical stamina you can call upon.
- Play for enjoyment – if you are not getting that, maybe you are in the wrong sport.

DRUGS AND SPORT

You may be tempted to boost performance and training by using steroids. These increase muscle bulk and, it is true, will take you to a higher level of power than you might achieve without them. Apart from being illegal (at least for professional athletes), the possible side-effects are mood changes (aggression and depression), acne and hair growth, and they also affect the liver.

SPORT AND RISK

The element of danger may well be what attracts you to a sport. However, there is a dividing line between a calculated risk and a death wish. Get your training from a recognized instructor, who will introduce you to the safety measures recommended for the sport, including how to use and maintain any equipment. Certain sports may be inadvisable for you, because of your build or stamina – this is something you can find out by trying sports and again by taking advice. If you are taking up a hazardous sport, you owe it to your family (especially if you have dependants) to get proper insurance that pays out in the event of serious injury or death. These are remote but not negligible hazards; during the years from late childhood to your late forties you are at far higher risk of injury through accidents at work or play than you are from serious medical conditions.

A LITTLE ABOUT SPORTS INJURIES

Many are simple sprains from over-stretching of tendons and muscles. The symptoms are pain, swelling and difficulty in use of that limb. Assuming serious injury is excluded (severe pain, deformity of a bone or joint, inability to bear weight or to use a limb) it is reasonable to treat yourself with RICE:

- Rest the limb, i.e. get off the sports pitch.
- Ice – cool the injury with ice, a pack of frozen peas or cold water; this reduces swelling.
- Compression – use a bandage or elasticated support, again to reduce swelling.
- Elevation – keep the limb raised to reduce swelling.

These simple remedies will limit the tissue damage from an injury and so speed up the process of healing. Later you may want to see a sports physiotherapist for further help to reduce pain and swelling and for supervised exercises to regain muscle power and joint movement.

EXERCISE – SOME MISCONCEPTIONS

It is dangerous

This myth derives from the few alarming reports of people dying during major sports events such as a marathon. The risk is estimated at 1 in 7,000 middle-aged people during a mass popular sports event such as a run. However, about half of those are already known to have some form of heart disease. Similar statistics show that the men at greatest risk are those who do not take regular exercise and then go in for something unusually vigorous.

So it is safer to make exercise a regular thing. If you are taking it up again after a long gap – six months or more – start cautiously with frequent pauses for rest. If you get chest pains, unusual breathlessness or feel faint – stop! See your doctor for a check-over.

Exercise is for the young

This is a complete myth. Regular exercise is of benefit whatever your age – you will feel the benefits after as little as two weeks and notice significant improvement in breathing and stamina after three months. As long as you take the common-sense approach above, you can enjoy exercise tailored to your age, with football and squash giving way to walking, swimming, dancing, golf and bowling as you get older. Aim for an exercise session two to three times a week – a brisk walk for a mile is ideal to start.

You have to wear the gear

Now this is a difficult one; should you invest in the designer stuff when you begin or wait until you know you are going to continue? This is not a frivolous question, because well-designed sports gear is comfortable and makes you feel bonded with others in the sport. We suggest you ask yourself three revealing questions:

- could you wear it outside the gym?
- can you look at yourself in a mirror without blushing?
- can your wife/girlfriend look at you without giggling?

If you answer 'yes' to two questions – go ahead. If less than that, examine your motives and bank balance carefully!

Smoking – the quit plan

You need not be a hero to give up smoking but you would be a fool not to. Here are some facts about smoking that smokers would rather not remember: 40 per cent of smokers will die from smoking-related diseases, including lung cancer, heart disease, strokes, arterial disease, chronic lung disease and cancer of the bladder, stomach, mouth and throat.

And here are some more things you might prefer to forget: smokers' skin ages faster; their children get more respiratory infection; their partners get lung cancer through passive smoking; smokers get indigestion and ulcers.

Do you need a cigarette within thirty minutes of waking up? If so, you are addicted and should make a serious effort to give up the weed. But even if you describe yourself as only a social smoker (having one or two of someone else's cigarettes down at the pub or at parties), you should also try to give up completely.

A QUIT PLAN
Your aim: to stop completely.

Step 1: preparation
- Convince yourself you want to stop smoking. Half hearted means half failed.
- List unpleasant aspects of smoking: cough, smells, bad breath, lack of money, burnt clothing and furniture.
- Remember friends, relatives and people you admire who have suffered from smoking-related illnesses.
- Consider why you smoke, when you smoke and what an alternative might be. For example, if you smoke to relax after a meal, a walk would be healthier; if you smoke while watching TV, try chewing gum instead.
- See if a colleague, friend or partner will quit with you.
- Prepare for a hard time for the first two to three weeks.
- Set the day: why not give up tomorrow? The sooner you stop the better. However, you are more likely to be successful if you choose a good time to stop – do not try when you know you are going to be under stress, if you are coming up to important exams, are about to make a major business presentation and so on.

Step 2: giving up
- Smoke your last cigarette and consign it to the bin together with any unused packs, matches and ash trays.
- Get in a supply of chewing gum or throat sweets.
- Arrange something to occupy you that first day – perhaps an outing or an absorbing task. Or go somewhere where smoking is prohibited, like the cinema or an art gallery. You will find it

easier if you avoid smoky environments during the first twenty-four hours.

- Reward yourself for achieving a cigarette-free day.

Step 3: staying off cigarettes
In some ways this is the hardest part.

- Avoid situations where you would have smoked until you feel confident about your will power.
- Develop alternative diversions.
- Each day, save the money you would have spent on cigarettes for a special goal.
- Try nicotine patches, gum or inhalators; they help many people.
- Know that the urge to smoke will pass.

Congratulations! You have made the biggest single step you can take for your future health. And if you tried and failed? Congratulations anyway; only a minority of smokers even take this step, and you can always try again. How about tomorrow?

Alcohol – a reducing plan

Do you crave a drink in the morning?
Do you regularly drink more than 35 units a week? (A unit is a glass of wine, a measure of spirits or half a pint of beer.)
Have you become impotent?
Are you or others worried about your drinking?
Are you not coping at work or home and see a drink as the answer?

If you answer yes to any of the above, you may well have an alcohol problem. Once you accept this, almost certainly you will be able to do something about it.

Alcohol is not inherently harmful. In fact alcohol is probably protective against heart disease, if limited to 2–3 units a day. Alcohol is a lubricant to business and social life. But it does get out of hand for about one in twenty men. This individual risks poor business performance, memory problems, gastric upsets, weight gain and poor nutrition. Plus high blood pressure, stroke, impotence, depression and having accidents. Your doctor may be able to show through blood tests any harmful effects on your liver.

STEPS TO SENSIBLE DRINKING

Step 1: you can do it

For most people the aim is sensible drinking, not complete abstinence.

- Think why you drink and where you drink.
- Keep a diary of alcohol consumption for a week.
- Think about other ways you could get relaxation such as yoga and massage – see the Appendix.
- Think how drink is affecting your health.

Step 2: setting limits

- Aim for no more than 21 units of alcohol a week.
- Ensure that at least two days a week are alcohol free
- Try soft drinks – you might like them.
- Be frank with your drinking partners; they will joke at the time, but one or two will be thinking 'Good man. If he can, I can'.

Step 3: seeing the benefits

Your sex drive will rise, your weight will fall, your indigestion vanish. Your work performance will improve. Blood tests will revert to normal. Most important of all, your self-esteem will return, because now you are achieving your full potential, without artificial aids.

Within reason, do not worry about the occasional binge, as long as you return to modest consumption afterwards. If you need more help, and serious drinkers may do, most towns have an alcohol advice centre listed in the phone book.

Sleep – and how to improve it

You are unusual if you can manage regularly on less than six hours of sleep a night. Most men need on average seven to eight hours, though we can cope with much less for a few nights.

What is sleep for? It is probably to do with organizing memory. Sleep and wakefulness are regulated by centres within the brain and though we can influence this, at times sleep will overwhelm us.

STAGES OF SLEEP

Broadly there are two types. A deep sleep associated with muscle relaxation, and a rapid eye movement (REM) sleep associated with flickering eye movement. REM sleep is when we dream; during that time a mechanism virtually paralyses our muscles so that the race, speech or caress we are dreaming about usually remains just a dream rather than an action.

DIFFICULTY GETTING TO SLEEP

Often physical factors are to blame such as eating too late, a too cold or hot room, an uncomfortable bed. Unfamiliar surroundings and noises will inhibit sleep. Otherwise worry is the main cause – thinking over the events of the day and tomorrow's tasks.

Action

If you worry over agendas, action plans and strategies, it is better to get up and perhaps write a sensible list of things to do tomorrow rather than let worry interfere with sleep. Make a routine for going to bed that psychologically prepares you. A bath, a small alcoholic drink or a warm drink, a book to read that engages but is not so exciting that you can't put it down.

Sex is an excellent hypnotic and beats sleeping pills most times.

Sleeping pills should be regarded as a last resort. Newer short-acting pills will give a good night's sleep without a hangover but responsible doctors will prescribe them only for a couple of weeks at a time. Do not take them after alcohol.

DIFFICULTY STAYING ASLEEP

Again, consider the physical factors given above. Heavy alcohol drinking will send you into a deep sleep initially, but often you will wake thirsty later. Worry is commonly to blame.

Action

Make your bed as comfortable as possible before going to sleep. If you have drunk a lot, drink at least a pint of water before retiring. Should you wake with worry which you cannot put out of your mind, it is better to get up and have a warm drink rather than lie there sweating.

EARLY WAKING

Regular early morning waking is often due to worry or even depression. You probably lie there in the early dawn contemplating a totally black and hopeless world.

Action

Do you have other features of depression such as poor concentration, inability to enjoy things, constant gloom, impotence, or excess drinking? Help is available either through counselling or with modern antidepressants (prescribed by your doctor) that will not inhibit your efficiency during the day.

Pollution protection plan

Here are some ways you can protect yourself, or remedy damage already done.

AIR

The problem: the air we breathe is contaminated with lead, sulphur, carbon monoxide, industrially generated dust or ash, and other impurities. A whole host of respiratory problems can result.

Protection: stopping breathing is obviously not an option, but there are things that you can do. Walk, cycle or take public transport – don't drive! The exercise will do your body good, and knowing that you are doing your bit for the planet will succour your mind and spirit. If you cycle, wear a helmet, and, if you are in a city, a mask as well.

WATER

The problem: our rivers and seas are contaminated with pesticides, insecticides, detergents, industrial effluents, oil spillage, sewage, ships' garbage and so on. Ingesting such contaminants can have negative effects throughout our bodies.

Protection: tap water in the developed world is safe but you may still want to filter your drinking water. Filters are available from leading pharmacies, hardware and department stores. Only drink bottled water in underdeveloped countries. When buying fish, bear in mind that pollutants particularly affect creatures living at the bottom of the river or ocean. This applies in particular to shellfish, which are notorious carriers of lead, cadmium, arsenic, and other heavy metals. This may be important in some parts of the world.

GROUND

The problem: pollutants from the air fall to earth, and pollutants from water leach into the soil. Agricultural sprays and pesticides are applied directly to the land, and rubbish is buried in it, sometimes in vast quantities. Again, ingesting such contaminants can have negative effects throughout our bodies.

Protection: try to buy organically grown food. Scrub or peel all root vegetables – potatoes, carrots, etc. If you live on, or near, a land-fill site, talk to your environmental health officer for additional advice.

LIGHT

The problem: when did you last stand in the pitch black, looking at the stars in all their glory? If you live in a city, it may have been a long time ago. Our cities are polluted by light from hundreds of thousands of homes and offices, from street lights and security lights. Light pollution can perhaps contribute to niggling mental health problems by subtly affecting our hormonal levels or causing energy imbalances.

Protection: if you live in a city, try to make regular night-time visits to an isolated place in the country. Seeing the stars at their brightest will refresh your sense of wonder at the universe, and your sense of smallness in it.

NOISE

The problem: again, the problem is greatest in the cities. If you live in the city, can you remember the last time you heard silence? No traffic noise, no car alarms, no aeroplanes overhead? Lack of access to silence, and to the noises of nature – birdsong and animal calls – can cause subtle negative effects throughout our bodies. Extended exposure to unwanted noise can cause hearing problems.

Protection: if your sleep is disrupted by noise pollution, have a cup of chamomile or vervain tea last thing at night, and buy some ear plugs – simple but effective. White noise can be used to block intrusive noise, but the machines to generate it are expensive, and not widely available.

REMEDYING DAMAGE

The following complementary therapies have a powerful anti-pollutant effect: auricular therapy, chakra balancing, reiki or therapeutic massage, ayurveda, Chinese and Western herbalism, Alexander Technique, yoga and T'ai chi/chi kung, meditation and breathing exercises, and massage. See the Appendix for further information.

Avoiding common infectious diseases

The germs causing these illnesses thrive because of their efficient strategies for transmission from host to host and survival within the host.

You do, however, enjoy certain advantages. You live in one of the healthiest societies ever known, with unprecedented protection against germs, thanks to general hygiene, vaccination and antibiotics. Easily available complementary remedies, such as the herb echinacea, can also help boost your immune system, to protect against infection.

Avoiding viral infection:

- have vaccinations against diphtheria, polio, measles, mumps etc.;
- have tetanus boosters every ten years.

Avoiding colds flu and coughs:

- use a handkerchief – sneezing spreads germs;
- wash your hands frequently – germs get transferred there from your nose;
- do not force yourself or others into work when you are coughing and sneezing;
- while you have a cold, do not share cups or utensils without washing them.

Avoiding gastric upsets:

- study what you are eating, the sell by date, the look, the smell;
- buy from outlets with a rapid turnover;
- keep your fridge organized and cold enough; store meat at the bottom so it cannot drip on to food below;
- keep cooked and raw food separate and use different utensils when preparing meat, fish and vegetables;
- thaw food thoroughly and cook according to instructions; always make sure hot food is thoroughly cooked;
- wash your hands frequently when handling food and after any visit to the toilet.

Avoiding travel hazards:

- know well in advance the hazards of the country you are visiting;
- get recommended vaccinations;
- if going to a malaria area, get advice on the pills to take – and take them;
- drink lots of fluids – but never tap water or ice unless you are confident of its safety.

Tests men should consider

Before having a health screen, review your lifestyle. If you smoke, drink heavily or take no exercise do you really need to hear more bad news?

NB: Tests marked with * are controversial, because there is current debate on how worthwhile they are or what to do about an abnormal result. Discuss the latest views with your doctor.

IN YOUR TWENTIES:

Check your weight every few months and seek advice if it is rapidly rising or falling.

Check your testicles regularly for lumps; this is the age for testicular cancer, which is curable if caught early.

Have your blood pressure checked at least once.

Have a urine test, for protein at least once (this may signify kidney problems).

IN YOUR THIRTIES AND FORTIES:

Weight: check as for your twenties.

Every three to five years, have checks on your blood pressure, cholesterol, and urine for protein and sugar (for kidney problems and diabetes).

IN YOUR FIFTIES AND ABOVE:

Weight: check as for your twenties.

Have an eye test for glaucoma.

Every three years, have your blood pressure, cholesterol and urine checked.

* Also every three years, have a prostate test i.e. a rectal examination of the prostate gland and a blood test of PSA (prostate specific antigen – a marker for prostate cancer).

* Get a sample of faeces analysed for blood, as an early marker of cancer of the bowel.

* Have an ECG (electrocardiogram – recording of the heart) while exercising. This is an early indicator of heart disease.

Depending on any symptoms you have, your GP may also advise chest X-ray, tests of anaemia, kidney or liver function, tests of respiratory function (breathing efficiency), testosterone (male sex hormone), or bone density (for osteoporosis).

Your family history is important. If parents or siblings had early heart trouble, get tested for cholesterol earlier. The same goes for glaucoma and bowel cancer.

MEDICALS AND CAREER DEVELOPMENT – DAVID'S STORY

Many companies now require potential employees to have pre-hiring medicals. David, a thirty-something computer analyst for a leading financial institution, is typical. 'Before I could join my new firm, I had to have a medical, to make sure nothing was wrong which would impede my ability to do my job – or which might kill me in the short term!'

You might argue that making a job offer conditional on passing a medical is an intrusion on personal liberty, but David was not worried: 'I was relaxed – the check-up provides information for yourself as well as the company, and if they find something wrong, you have a chance to act. You are given general lifestyle advice, which is helpful. For me, the results were all reassuring – I came out after my allotted hour and a half feeling much more confident about my health than when I went in.'

So what tests did David actually have? First of all, he was given an assessment of his general physical condition: 'A doctor gave me a once-over, including an examination of my goolies, and I was given advice about self-examination to check for possible testicular cancer. Next I was measured, and weighed, and callipers were used to determine my body fat level. I learned that weight itself is not a reliable indicator of physical condition, it's the amount of fat that's important. Results showed my body fat level was within the ideal range, so I need only concern myself with keeping it there.'

Next David's lungs were tested, for lung volumes – the amount of air going in and out of them – the condition of the airways, and for function during exercise. David had to put on a facemask and blow in and out of a machine, which automatically monitored the level of gases in his breath. Meanwhile he was peddling furiously on an exercise bike.

Lung volumes can be affected by smoking, asthma or pollution. David's lung volumes were within normal limits, showing no evidence of loss from these sources, but for some this test can be the first indication that they are asthmatic. The condition of the airways affects the ability of the lung linings to transfer oxygen into the blood. Again, this was normal for David.

Breathing patterns during exercise and the way in which the body is using fuel jointly give a picture of metabolism, which shows how well the body is equipped to cope with the demands of your lifestyle. (See page 28 for a fuller explanation.)

After monitoring his fuel use, David's health assessment team was able to give specific advice about exercise: 'I already knew that the exercise which is most effective in improving cardiovascular fitness is aerobic exercise, and that I ought to be maintaining a moderate exercise rate for twenty-five to thirty minutes two to three times a week. I knew it, but I didn't act on it, although I thought I was fit. Worryingly, my metabolism tests showed an early reliance on anaerobic work, suggesting my metabolism was unable to cope with steady exertion. I needed more aerobic training. As a result of the fitness test, I began to go jogging twice weekly after work – something I hadn't done for years and came to look forward to. Jogging is good aerobic exercise, and ideal for me because it can be done anytime, anywhere, without any special facilities. I now also try to swim once a week.'

If, like David, you decide to take up jogging, invest in a well-designed pair of trainers, and try to run on soft surfaces, such as grass. These measures will reduce stress on your knees.

After the lung tests, David's heart and circulatory system were also examined. He was strapped up to an ECG machine, which measures electrical signals from the heart, while still pedalling energetically on his bike. Two readings gave an indication of his heart's performance during exercise. They showed the increase in his pulse rate, and the efficiency of his heart in delivering oxygen to his muscles. Two other readings gave an indication of his arterial blood pressure, one measuring the highest blood pressure during heartbeat, the other the lowest.

Assessing the performance of the heart during exercise may reveal problems long before they are apparent on tests at rest, or give symptoms such as chest pain. The results were collated to give David a summary of risk factors for the future development of coronary heart disease. 'My results indicated that my heart and circulation have an average level of efficiency in delivering oxygen to my muscles and that my blood pressure was well controlled throughout exercise. I was told how to take steps to keep risk factors as low as possible – for me, these mainly related to healthy eating and keeping fit – I don't smoke, but if I did, I know they would have told me to try to quit.'

David had thorough eye tests that confirmed he is short-sighted, and also revealed he has a slight astigmatism. 'My distance vision and near vision were both tested, as well as my colour perception, field of vision and VDU vision – a measure of how well my eyes cope with staring at computer screens all day! Wearing my glasses, my visual acuity was average or above at all distances, showing they are doing a perfectly good job.'

The pressure inside both David's eyes was also measured, using a special machine which blows air on to the surface of the eye. Intra-ocular pressure, as it is called, gives an indication of glaucoma risk. Glaucoma is a disease of the eyes where increased pressure gradually causes loss of sight – it is frequently hereditary. For all of us, visual function can change rapidly, and you are advised to have regular check-ups, perhaps every two years, especially if you have a family history of eye problems.

Naturally David had to provide a urine sample – 'not much fun to pee to order, but I managed it!' His sample was tested for acidity, and for substances whose presence would have indicated some kidney or metabolic problem. Testing for drug residues was not part of the standard package, although David is used to the possibility of random drug tests at work – 'anybody can be tested, anytime, especially if they give any cause for suspicion.'

Blood was taken, for instant analysis. 'Giving a blood sample was the only bit I really didn't enjoy – they seemed to come at me with a huge needle. I wasn't happy.' David's blood was subjected to twenty-two different tests. In summary, they were for the following:

- Lipid levels (especially cholesterol) – raised levels indicate increased risk of heart and circulatory disease.
- Liver function – to look for alcohol-associated impairment, as well as more general indicators. David, who regards his alcohol

intake as minimal, was told that his liver function tests reflected a degree of over-work by his liver. He was advised to reduce his alcohol intake and have his blood checked again in three months.

- Kidney function – to look for inefficiency of the kidneys and increased risk of kidney stone formation.
- Glucose levels – increased levels may indicate diabetes.
- Uric acid – raised levels indicate risk of gout.
- Anaemia – low levels of haemoglobin, the oxygen-carrying pigment in the blood, indicate anaemia, possibly due to iron deficiency.
- Blood cells – the balance of values between the various blood cells can give early warning of a range of problems, or indicate the cause of a known problem.

There was no specific HIV test. David had assumed that there would be, and since he had already had to have one in order to get life insurance he wasn't worried about the prospect. But in fact, his medical included a much more general test of defence and inflammatory system activation. If the test gives a reading over 20, there may be something major wrong, although the test alone cannot reveal what it is – that requires further diagnosis. Fortunately for David, his reading was a healthy 1 – he had to wait a few days for the result, as in this case immediate analysis is not possible.

Health assessment results are presented in ways which can be easily understood. This is usually a simple graph, shaded to show how the person's results compare with those of people of the same sex, and similar age. Did David refer back to these results? Did he act on the advice he was given? 'Sure. I found the graphs very useful, and I came away with a sheaf of papers on testicular self-examination, exercise, heart health, healthy eating, etc. I read them all, in conjunction with my results, and took appropriate action. For example, I did cut down on my alcohol intake, although I haven't had the blood test repeated yet. And I did change my exercise programme.'

What about follow-up? Does his firm insist on regular check-ups? Indeed is promotion dependent on it? If not, would he in any case go back? 'The company doesn't insist on employees taking regular medicals once they've been hired, but it offers them the chance every two years. I'll certainly take them up on the offer – it's only sensible. What's more, I was so impressed by the screening that I've booked my wife in for a health assessment – at my own expense.'

Life insurance and tests for HIV/AIDS/hepatitis

Life insurance is a carefully calculated bet by the insurance company on your chances of surviving and them having to pay out. They assess that risk from life tables; these are life expectancies for people with all sorts of risk factor. You can imagine the list: being overweight, smoking, drinking, with a poor family history of illness. Certain occupations carry high risk – for example, publicans and journalists because some adverse lifestyle aspects (like drinking alcohol) attaches to their occupation.

THE LIFE INSURANCE QUESTIONNAIRE

This is designed to highlight risk factors as listed above. The companies are greatly interested in the health of your parents and siblings because this is a major influence on your likely health. Breeding is all. But smoking, drinking and self-abuse through drugs or self-neglect are major additional risks in your hands.

People often worry about revealing psychological problems. Insurers generally ignore these if they occur within understandable contexts – such as depression at the time of divorce or job loss. They look seriously on recurrent problems and any history of self-harm.

THE LIFE INSURANCE EXAMINATION

Companies are most interested in your height/weight ratio, blood pressure and analysis of urine for sugar or protein. Your heart is checked, your abdomen felt, your nervous system tested and your testicles prodded. Also your ears, eyes and mouth are examined and your back checked. These examinations rarely turn up a major surprise.

Blood tests

It is becoming routine to have HIV tests if you are taking out high insurance cover. The tests will show if you have contracted the virus, though not within the last three months, the time it takes for the test to go positive. Some companies ask for tests of hepatitis B and C. These are usually transmitted by homosexual sex or intravenous drug use (though not invariably) and carry a significant risk of later liver trouble. They are also a reflection on lifestyle.

What happens about abnormal results?

The examining doctor, even if he or she is your regular doctor, is working for the insurance company and is contractually bound not to reveal any results to you. The first you will know is if the insurance is turned down or is loaded, i.e. you have to pay an extra premium reflecting extra risk. Companies will reveal the reasons, but only through your own doctor.

ALTERNATIVE CHECK-UPS

If you are looking for alternatives to the standard health checks, why not try iridology, kirlian photography or kinesiology? All are primarily diagnostic therapies.

Iridology

Iridologists links the state of the iris of your eyes to your health and to potential physical or psychological problems.

Kirlian photography

This is based on the theory that we are all electrical beings, and that electrical energy can be photographed and analysed to determine the state of your health.

Kinesiology

Practitioners believe that the study of movement will reveal your physical, emotional and mental state of health.

See the Appendix for further details of each of these therapies.

Accidents and how to avoid them

Accidents are a major cause of avoidable ill-health, injury and death. Men are at significantly greater risk than women, and they are the most common cause of male death under thirty. Here are some suggestions for protecting yourself. They might seem obvious, but every day men ignore them, and every day men and their dependants suffer as a result. If you are tempted to say, 'That's just common sense!' pause to ask yourself whether you actually follow the advice all the time.

ON THE ROAD

Nearly 50 per cent of deaths in men under thirty are caused by road traffic accidents, and men are at significantly greater risk than women. In 1995 2,541 men were killed in road traffic accidents in Britain, compared to 1,080 women; and 29,360 men were seriously injured, compared to 16,160 women. Head injuries form a large proportion of these statistics, and brain damage is common.

BRAIN DAMAGE

Terrible damage can be inflicted on the brain when a head travelling at high speed is suddenly decelerated by striking something. In such circumstances the soft, jelly-like brain continues to travel forwards at the original speed and is smashed against the front inside of the skull. It then swings back and is smashed against the inside of the back of the skull. The injuries which result can have devastating effects...loss of the ability to speak, paralysis, incontinence, long-term visual disturbance, etc.

What you can do

- Have you been driving for under two years? Lack of experience is a major cause of accidents among new drivers – over-confidence can kill.
- Never drink and drive. Similarly, never allow yourself to be driven by someone who has been drinking. The same goes for taking drugs. Alcohol, and to a lesser extent drugs, are significant factors in road traffic accidents.

- Never use a mobile phone while driving. Do not take both hands off the wheel, and your eyes off the road, to eat a sandwich, flick through a map, etc.
- Always wear your seat belt. Ensure that your passengers are wearing theirs.
- Whatever the temptations, try not to exceed the speed limit. Try to drive sensibly, under all conditions. It is common to see powerful cars and motorcycles driven in a stupid fashion. In fog and rain, there are frequently pile-ups caused by drivers ignoring all the hazard signs. If you are a speed-merchant, re-read the notes about the effect of sudden deceleration on the brain.
- Before buying a new car, think about its safety features, as well as power and design. Does your chosen car have air-bags? Does it have side-impact bars? Safety might seem dull, but it saves lives.
- If you cycle, always wear a helmet. Be safe, be seen; wear bright colours or fluorescent clothing during the day, and reflective clothing at night.

IN THE HOME

Accidents in the home are the second most common cause of death and injury by accident, after road traffic accidents. They include accidental poisoning, accidental falls, accidents caused by fire, electrocutions, etc.

What you can do

- Have a smoke alarm fitted, and check it about once a month. Make sure you know how to get out of your house in a fire. Fit a wall-mounted fire extinguisher in your kitchen. Beware of the chip pan. Never fill it more than a third with oil, and never leave it unattended. Do not let curtains, or other fabrics, dangle near open fires, candles or any other flames.
- Keep household cleaning fluids away from food, in a separate, locked cupboard. Keep medicines in a locked cabinet. Keep garden chemicals locked away, preferably in their original containers. Never decant them into old lemonade or drinks bottles.
- DIY can be dangerous. Check your ladder is in good condition, and when you use it, ask a helper to stand at the bottom to hold it steady. If you use dangerous tools at home – a chain saw, for

example – make sure you wear all the relevant protective clothing, goggles and masks. Always use your protective gear, even if the task will only take a couple of minutes.

- Kitchens, bathrooms and stairs are particularly dangerous areas of the house. Check yours for potential hazards. Is the lighting adequate? Are the banisters wobbly? Are there any loose wires? Are items such as knives safely stowed? Do you have something to hold as you climb in and out of the bath?

- Be careful not to plug too many appliances into one electrical socket. Check wires for signs of fraying; do not let flexes and cables overhang work-surfaces.

ON THE PLAYING FIELD

More than 1 million people a year require hospital treatment for sporting injuries. If you pursue extreme sports, like hang-gliding, paragliding or sports diving, then you will know the risks, and be aware of precautions to lessen them. But less extreme sports carry risk too, and amateurs are at greater risk than professionals. Sprains, breaks and fractures are all too common. Even relatively minor injuries can have a dramatic effect on your life. A snapped knee tendon might require a couple of months of intensive pre-operative physiotherapy, several reconstructive operations, and then months more post-operative physiotherapy. It is worth taking precautions.

What you can do

- Do not forget to do your stretching and warm-up exercises before you start any type of sporting session, and remember to do your cooling down exercises afterwards.

- Always make sure you have, and use, adequate footwear and protective gear relevant to your sport. Demand that your club or gym takes adequate protective measures. For example, if you play rugby, make sure your club pads the posts.

- Does your club or gym have first-aid facilities? Is there a group of named first-aiders? Make sure you know the basics of first aid.

- Think about taking out specialist insurance in case the worst happens. Many leading health insurers have begun to realize the potential of the market among amateur sportsmen, and can arrange specialist cover.

AT WORK

In 1995–96, 183 men were killed in accidents at work, compared to nine women. Over 11,500 men suffered major injuries, and 92,383 were involved in accidents causing them to take more than three days off work. The four most risky sectors are construction, manufacturing, agriculture and, surprisingly, services. The law requires your employer to protect your health and safety at work – always tell your supervisor, or personnel department, if you have any concerns about this.

What you can do

- Protect your back. Before lifting or moving any load, stop and think. Correct lifting techniques (see page 62) cannot prevent all back injuries – consider the use of handling equipment, like a trolley or hoist, instead.
- Protect your hands and arms. Jobs which involve rapid, repetitive, unnatural movements may cause pain or swelling here. Check that your workstation is efficiently laid out, with all your equipment in easy reach. Your desk and chair should be at a comfortable height for you, and equipment should be comfortable to use, with any vibration kept to a minimum. Pace your work, and try to switch to other tasks whenever you can.
- Protect your skin. At work the areas of skin most at risk are on the hands, forearms and legs above footwear. If you work with known contaminants, wear protective clothing, such as gloves and aprons. Try not to touch harmful substances – apply them with a brush, for instance. Wash contaminated skin if it comes into contact with harmful substances; use purpose-made cleansers to remove oil or grease. If you work outside, be careful not to get too much exposure to the sun.
- Protect your lungs – asbestos is carcinogenic. Construction and building maintenance workers can be exposed to asbestos dust without realizing it. If you discover any material or dust which you suspect contains asbestos, stop work and get advice. If you are working with other dangerous substances, make sure you are aware of control measures, and that any protective clothing is in good condition. Do not store gloves inside respirator helmets.

- Protect your hearing – noise can be a problem in many jobs. Use any noise control equipment provided; never remove from a machine any noise control devices; wear ear protectors if there is a risk to your hearing, and keep them in good condition – replace the muffs regularly.
- Protect your mental health – stress is often work-related. Possible factors include inappropriate work demands, lack of control over your work, not enough support and poor working relationships. Talk over your problem with someone you trust.

The real chiller killers – common male illnesses

Though everyone dies, men tend to die sooner and younger than women. This is a price paid for being male, because male hormones increase the risk of heart disease and prostate cancer. But there are steps you can take to reduce your natural risk to the minimum.

CORONARY HEART DISEASE

If the heart's own blood supply furs up (atherosclerosis) eventually you will develop heart disease. Atherosclerosis refers to a sludgy deposit of cholesterol and blood clots on the walls of arteries.

WHAT IS THE RISK?

Coronary artery disease as heart attacks or heart failure is the biggest single cause of death in the UK. Of those 150,000 deaths a year 55 per cent are men. One third of men over sixty-five have coronary artery disease in some form.

HOW DO I RECOGNIZE IT?

Angina

This is pain in the chest on exercise that goes after a few minutes rest. Often the pain radiates up the neck or down the left arm. There are many other causes of chest pain, but angina is the one to have checked out.

Failing heart

You will get breathless easily and feel unusually tired. Because of fluid retention, your ankles may swell and you may get breathless lying flat at night as fluid accumulates on the lungs.

Heart attack

A crushing severe pain over the breastbone, with breathlessness and collapse of blood pressure. You do not want this to be your first hint of heart trouble.

WHAT CAN BE DONE?

Prevention

Stop smoking. Any smoking is bad, but having more than twenty cigarettes a day at least triples your risk of heart trouble. Check your cholesterol, especially if you have a family history of heart trouble. Your doctor will advise how low your cholesterol should be. Take regular exercise – just two or three brisk walks a week of a mile or so are sufficient, but take more if you can manage it. Reduce your weight (if you have excess weight to lose), and if you have raised blood pressure get it treated. Also, a regular alcohol intake (two or three glasses of wine a day or one or two pints of beer) appears protective against heart disease, though excess leads to its own problems (see page 33).

Treatment

There are many drugs to control angina, heart failure, high blood pressure and cholesterol. You may need angiography (X-rays showing the state of your coronary arteries) and replacement of the affected arteries (coronary artery bypass grafting). If you have a heart attack, get to hospital immediately for treatment. Afterwards you may be advised to take aspirin and other drugs to protect your heart.

STROKE

This is when an artery in the brain ruptures or becomes blocked with a blood clot.

WHAT IS THE RISK?

In the UK there are about 100,000 major strokes a year and many minor ones. Below the age of fifty-five there is a less than 1 in 1,000 annual risk but this rises to 10 in 1,000 annual risk at age seventy-five. Men are at slightly greater risk at all ages except in the eighties. Although 20 per cent of victims die within a month, 50 per cent of survivors make an eventual full recovery.

HOW TO RECOGNIZE IT
The symptoms are sudden loss of use of an arm or leg, slurred speech, loss of vision and confusion. In the worst strokes there is sudden collapse and unconsciousness. Recovery may take hours or many months.

WHAT CAN BE DONE?
Prevention
The greatest risk is from high blood pressure; have a check every few years. There is an increased risk if you smoke, have diabetes, heart disease or irregular heart rhythms. Taking a low dose of aspirin every day may prevent stroke but it is not suitable for everyone. See your doctor for advice.

Treatment
You need a brain scan to determine the type of stroke and the appropriate treatment. A few strokes are treatable by surgery on the diseased artery. Most are treated by controlling high blood pressure, rehabilitation therapy and aspirin if suitable for you.

MALE CANCERS

Prostate cancer
The prostate gland lies in the perineum between the root of the penis and the anus; it encircles the urethra, near the outlet from the bladder.

WHAT IS THE RISK?
Prostate cancer is the second most common cancer in men, after lung cancer, and causes over 9,000 deaths a year. It mainly affects men above sixty-five; just 2 per cent of cases occur below age fifty-five, and 16 per cent below sixty-five.

HOW TO RECOGNIZE IT

Prostate cancer causes the same symptoms as benign overgrowth of the prostate gland: difficulty in passing urine, a poor stream, a need to pass small amounts day and night. Without investigation it is impossible to tell benign prostate trouble from prostate cancer.

WHAT CAN BE DONE?
Prevention

There is no agreed method of detecting prostate cancer early. Some specialists recommend all men above fifty to fifty-five to have an annual rectal examination of their prostate gland and a blood test called PSA (prostate specific antigen), though there is no agreement at the time of writing about what to do in the case of an abnormal result.

Treatment

Several drugs (including cyproterone and goserelin) reduce the activity of the cancer. Other treatment is with radiotherapy and surgical removal of the gland. Aggressive treatment of early cancer improves survival but risks side-effects of impotence and incontinence of urine. This is a rapidly changing field; you should seek up-to-date advice from your doctor.

Cancer of the testicle

WHAT IS THE RISK?

This is the commonest cancer in men in their twenties and thirties, affecting 1,250 men a year. If treated early it is entirely curable.

HOW TO RECOGNIZE IT

There is a lump in the testicle, which feels hard and heavy.

WHAT CAN BE DONE?
Prevention

Men of all ages, especially in their twenties and thirties, should regularly check their testicles for lumps. See a doctor about anything which feels odd or painful. There is a slightly higher risk if you had undescended testicles in childhood.

Treatment
You will need radiotherapy, chemotherapy and possibly removal of the affected testicle. The outlook is excellent.

Breast cancer
WHAT IS THE RISK?
This rare cancer affects under 200 men a year.

HOW TO RECOGNIZE IT
It causes a lump in the breast or a discharge from the nipple.

WHAT CAN BE DONE
The treatment is the same as in women – a combination of radiotherapy, surgery and chemotherapy.

Lung cancer
WHAT IS THE RISK?
More men die from lung cancer than any other form of cancer – 25,000 a year as against 12,500 women. It is almost always self-inflicted through smoking. A small number of lung cancers are caused by passive smoking, exposure to asbestos, industrial dusts or chance.

HOW TO RECOGNIZE IT?
Anyone, but especially smokers, should take seriously a persistent cough, pain over one lung and the slightest hint of coughing blood. Other warnings might be recurrent chest infections and weight loss.

WHAT CAN BE DONE?
Prevention
If you are going to act on only one piece of advice in this book, make it giving up smoking. In quitting, you will reduce your risks not only of lung cancer but heart disease, stomach cancer, arterial disease and stroke. Avoid passive smoking and wear protective clothes and masks if you work in a polluted environment.

Treatment
Unfortunately, lung cancer is rarely curable; only 4–8 per cent of sufferers survive for five years. Chemotherapy and radiotherapy can help reduce symptoms such as pain and breathlessness.

Cancer of the gastrointestinal tract (gullet, stomach, bowel and pancreas)

WHAT IS THE RISK?

Together these are the commonest group of cancers, especially in the sixties onwards but they do occur before then. Cancer of the colon or rectum is the third most common cancer in men, causing about 8,500 deaths a year. It is more likely if there is a family history of bowel cancer or in sufferers of ulcerative colitis. Cancer of the pancreas causes 8,000 deaths a year, especially in smokers and diabetics. Cancer of the gullet or stomach affect an older age group and are more common in smokers.

HOW TO RECOGNIZE IT

The symptoms of bowel cancer are a change in bowel habit – for example, unusual constipation or persistent diarrhoea or blood in the motions. Cancer of the gullet causes difficulty swallowing. Stomach cancer begins as persistent indigestion, upper abdominal pain and loss of appetite, possibly with vomiting of blood. Pain or weight loss are features of more advanced disease of any of the above. Cancer of the pancreas is notoriously difficult to diagnose early; it may cause a vague abdominal pain, jaundice and weight loss.

WHAT CAN BE DONE?

Prevention

See a doctor if your bowel habit alters for more than two weeks without some good reason. Always take seriously any difficulty in swallowing. Indigestion beginning for the first time above the age of forty-five should be investigated, even though stomach cancer is relatively uncommon until the sixties. Never ignore persistent weight loss and loss of appetite.

Treatment

Surgical removal of early bowel and stomach cancers gives excellent long-term results; this is why you should not delay in having suspicious symptoms investigated. The outlook for cancer of the gullet and pancreas is much poorer; even so much can be done to relieve discomfort.

Cancer – all other types

WHAT IS THE RISK?

Other cancers include leukaemia (cancer of the bone marrow), lymphoma (cancer of the lymph nodes e.g. Hodgkin's disease), and bone cancers. None of these is especially common but taken together they add up to large numbers. Skin cancer is much more common.

HOW TO RECOGNIZE IT

Do not ignore:

- new and persistent lumps especially around the neck;
- localized pains, e.g. over a bone or gland;
- skin blemishes that bleed, itch, grow or turn black;
- unusual tiredness.

WHAT CAN BE DONE?

Many of the above cancers are curable if caught early, especially skin cancer. It is a large part of a doctor's work to assess lumps, pains and unusual symptoms. They will not feel you are making a fuss about nothing so you should not feel embarrassed about seeing a doctor when a symptom is worrying you.

SUICIDE

Deliberately killing yourself is the ultimate response to overwhelming despair.

WHAT IS THE RISK?

In the UK 4,000–4,500 people commit suicide each year, over two thirds of whom are men. Factors increasing the risk are social isolation, alcoholism, drug abuse, depression, serious physical or psychiatric illness.

HOW TO RECOGNIZE A PROBLEM

Seek professional help if you are getting increasingly depressed and see no point in living. Other symptoms include poor sleep, early-morning waking and worrying, lack of concentration, loss of appetite, loss of any enjoyment in life and finding yourself crying.

WHAT CAN BE DONE?
Prevention
Depression may be both an illness and a reaction to adverse life events. Either way it is not a sign of weakness to admit to being depressed. Early counselling and support will prevent you sliding into a state of despair, so talk to people about how you feel, rather than turning to drink, drugs or isolation.

Treatment
This includes counselling, suicide helplines like the Samaritans (Linkline: 0345 909090, or look in the phone book for local branches). Modern antidepressants are effective, non-addictive and have few side-effects.

LIVING WITH A HEALTH PROBLEM

Long-term, chronic health problems will affect many different areas of your life – career, family, and social activities. Here are some strategies for lessening your risk, reducing the severity of problems, managing during a crisis, and coping afterwards.

ASTHMA

In asthma, the diameter of the small airways in the lungs narrows severely, making breathing difficult.

Risk: 10–15 per cent of the population suffers asthma – men and women are at equal risk. In young adults, just 1 death per 100,000 a year is a attributable to asthma. In the over sixty-fives, asthma causes approximately 2,000 deaths a year. Asthma tends to run in families, and can be linked to eczema. Diet, smoking and pollution may all aggravate the symptoms.

Recognition: symptoms are a recurrent wheeze, a persistent cough, especially one brought on by changes in temperature, or which is worse at night, or is made worse by exercise, breathlessness, and having to make an effort to breathe. During an asthmatic attack the victim will gasp for air, and may turn blue from lack of oxygen.

Doctors investigate these symptoms using a device to test how efficiently you can breathe out, chest X-rays, and sometimes, tests for allergies.

Plan A: self-help and prevention

- Avoid contact with trigger factors, such as animal fur or dust. Use pillows filled with man-made fibres, not feathers. Other potential triggers include chocolate, convenience foods containing colourings or preservatives, peanuts and shellfish.
- Self-promoting panic can worsen an asthma attack. To reduce this possibility, explore relaxation and breathing techniques, such as those described on page 148.
- If a mild attack of wheezing has been sparked by breathing very cold air, it may help to sip a warm drink, in relaxed surroundings.
- If breathing is difficult do not lie down. Sit leaning slightly forwards with your elbows resting on the back of a chair. Try to relax, and to breathe evenly and gently. Concentrate on slowly expanding your chest. If breathlessness persists, seek medical help.

Plan B: treatment

Your GP will prescribe bronchodilators (which work by relaxing the muscles surrounding the airways, thus enabling them to open up) and often steroids too. Drugs can be delivered via puffers (inhalers), nebulizers, which generate a fine cloud of gas, or by mouth. It is very important that you maintain the treatment regime recommended by your doctor, but, in addition, you might want to explore complementary approaches. Tell your doctor what you are doing, and check that your chosen practitioner is registered with an appropriate regulatory body, and is experienced in treating asthma. You should not attempt to self-prescribe complementary drugs for asthma.

For more about self-help relaxation techniques, see Appendix.

DIABETES

In diabetes, there is too much sugar in the bloodstream. The level of blood sugar is linked to the level of the hormone insulin, which is made by the pancreas. Without insulin, sugar is not absorbed by the body. In the most serious form of diabetes, which usually appears at under age forty, there is a decrease in the amount of insulin made by the body, which if left untreated leads to rapid and serious ill-health, coma and death. Less dramatic symptoms appear in older people, who continue to manufacture normal amounts of insulin, but who have built up a resistance to its effects.

Risk: about 2 per cent of Europeans, and those of European descent, are diabetic. Excluding temporary diabetes during pregnancy, men and women are at equal risk. Obesity is a risk factor for late onset diabetes. Your genetic inheritance is important. Diabetes is commoner in some population groups than in others – for instance, it is five times more common in those from south-east Asia, than in Europeans. Damage to the pancreas – perhaps from alcohol-related diseases – can lead to diabetes.

Recognition: you find you are passing unusually large quantities of urine, night and day. As a result of losing all this fluid, you feel constantly thirsty. You may notice that you are rapidly losing weight. However, many people who develop late onset diabetes are overweight, and continue to gain weight. You will find that you are constantly tired, since your body cannot access energy locked up in blood sugar. Grazes and scratches become infected very easily because bacteria are taking advantage of your high blood sugar levels. Your vision may become blurred, and your fingers and toes may tingle, or become numb.

Doctors use urine tests to check for sugar in the urine, and blood tests to see if your blood contains very high levels of sugar. If you are diagnosed as diabetic, you will be given a general physical examination, to see if the disease has caused any damage to your body. The commonest forms of damage are to the eyes (diabetes is the commonest cause of blindness in the UK), widespread arterial disease, which makes you especially prone to ulcers of the feet, kidney damage and nerve damage, which can sometimes lead to impotence.

Plan A: self-help and prevention

It is important to follow any treatment regime prescribed by your doctor, but there is much you can do to help keep your condition under control.

- Diet – you will be asked to avoid refined sugars, and there are recommended levels for protein and fat. Otherwise you should be able to follow a fairly normal diet, including plenty of wholefoods, fruit and vegetables. A dietitian will tailor a diet to suit your needs.

- Diet supplements – whichever type of diabetes you have, it might be worth supplementing your vitamin E intake. For late onset diabetes, you could consider B vitamins, and the minerals zinc, chromium and magnesium. Discuss supplementation with your doctor, before you begin, and get detailed advice from a dietitian, naturopath or nutritional therapist.
- Exercise – do incorporate exercise into your weekly routine. Make sure it is something you enjoy, not something you have to force yourself to do.
- Have regular chiropody. Badly clipped toe-nails are dangerous for diabetics, because this is where ulcers and infections begin.
- Have annual eye checks – early eye problems can be treated with laser treatment.
- Learn a stress-reducing relaxation technique (see Appendix).
- If on medication, wear a medic alert bracelet at all times.

Plan B: treatment

Diet alone may be enough to control mild late onset diabetes, or you may be able to take tablets. Sometimes there is no substitute for insulin delivered by self-administered daily injections – clever, pen-like devices make this easy and pain free. You will be taught to self-inject by a specially trained diabetic nurse. It is important to monitor your control; you can do this at home using simple kits to test your urine or blood for sugar. At least once a year you will need a general physical examination and more sophisticated blood tests at a diabetic clinic.

Complementary approaches cannot cure diabetes, and should never be used as an alternative to orthodox medicine. However, autogenic training could help you keep the condition under control. It allows mind and body to rebalance themselves. Hormone levels rise and fall according to the system's needs. Severe insulin controlled diabetes will not respond, but in combination with dietary control, good results can be achieved for maturity onset diabetes.

BACK PAIN

Back pain is usually caused by one of the following: over-strain to the muscles in the back; damage to the ligaments supporting the spine; or damage to the small vertebral joints (discs). Contrary to popular opinion, discs, which are located between the vertebrae and act as shock absorbers, do not slip. Rather they contain a gelatinous core, surround by a fibrous ring, and with age, or injury, the ring ruptures, enabling the gel to spill out and press on nerves radiating from the spinal cord.

Risk: back pain affects 75 per cent of people at some time or another. There is a doubled risk for people in jobs involving lifting, carrying and bending, such as farm labourers, warehouse men or car mechanics. Sportsmen who enjoy contact sports are at increased risk of back pain. About 1 per cent of the population suffers a so-called slipped disc each year, most of them aged between twenty-five and forty-five. There is only a 10 per cent risk of back pain being a symptom of serious, underlying disease – your doctor will advise you if this is the case.

Recognition: this is easy enough! Pain often seems to radiate down the leg (sciatica), and you may experience tingling, or numbness down your leg. It may not be possible for you to stand straight, or to stand at all. If you get a numb bum, tell your doctor; this can be a symptom that the nerves at the base of your spine are being squashed, and you need immediate investigation.

Doctors test the degree of restriction in your movement with a variety of physical stretching and bending tests. They will also test your reflexes, by tapping your knees and ankles, and running a fine point up and down the soles of your feet. This enables them to judge whether there is pressure on the nerves into your legs, and if so, where it is. More sophisticated, but less frequently used, investigations include CT (computed tomography) and MRI (magnetic resonance imaging) scans. These show the structure of the back in greater detail than X-rays.

Plan A: self-help and prevention

- Think about how you lift things – especially heavy or awkward objects. Stand close to anything you need to lift, gain a good grip and secure your foothold. Bend your knees, lift without jerking, and keep your back straight. Do not twist or stoop when you put the object down. If you need help, ask for it or, even better, use a hoist or trolley.
- Think about your posture. If you need advice ask your GP to refer you to a physiotherapist, or consult a teacher of the Alexander Technique.

- If you sit at a computer screen all day, demand a chair which supports your back. Experiment with different chairs, and different heights for your desk. Make sure you do not have to bend your neck to look at your computer screen – most of us keep our screens too low. When you are at the keyboard, try to keep your wrists flat, at ninety degrees to your body.
- Except during acute attacks, continue to take exercise which stretches your back – swimming and brisk walking are both excellent forms of exercise for back-pain sufferers.

Plan B: treatment

During an acute attack, you will have no alternative but to rest, since your body will not let you do otherwise. Take simple painkillers such as paracetamol or ibuprofen – this contains a non-steroidal, anti-inflammatory drug. If muscle spasm is a problem, your GP may prescribe a muscle relaxant.

Surgery is reserved for the very few cases where scans have shown disc or bone damage. Surgeons may either remove a disc, to release pressure on nerves, or fuse bones in the spine, so nerves are no longer stretched when you bend.

Manipulative therapies are often helpful. Massage, osteopathy and chiropractic are the best known. Rolfing and Hellerwork can also be beneficial; both work on the principle that a structurally misaligned body experiences gravity as stressful, so movement and flexibility are limited. The aim is to realign the body so that it experiences gravity as a supporting force, is flexible and moves easily.

JOINT AND MUSCLE PAIN

Joint and muscle pain have a great variety of causes; injury and strain are particular problems for sportsmen. Once we hit thirty, our joints start to show signs of wear and tear (arthritis). Occasionally, rheumatoid arthritis, which is a disease involving the immune system, can also be a cause.

Risk: most sportsmen suffer joint or muscle pain at some point, as do people with jobs involving heavy lifting. About 20 per cent of white people complain of arthritis, but it is relatively uncommon in blacks. Obesity is a risk factor. In all ethnic groups, 2–3 per cent of people suffer rheumatoid arthritis, but it is three times as common in women than in men – plus there is a genetic element in the risk.

Recognition: joint and muscle pain are easy enough to recognize. If the cause is not obvious, your doctor might order an X-ray, or blood tests.

Plan A: self-help and prevention

See pages 49 and 50 for advice on minimizing risk from sports injuries, and from injuries to your hands and arms at work.

- If you are overweight, try to shed a few pounds, and eat healthily.
- Keep active, but try not to put jarring stresses on joints. Jogging is not a good idea, but if you must jog, make sure you have suitable footwear. Walking and swimming are excellent alternatives.
- Consider taking cod-liver oil, which lubricates joints.

Plan B: treatment

If arthritis or rheumatoid arthritis is the problem, a range of drugs is available, and surgery is sometimes necessary. However, for relatively young, otherwise fit men, physiotherapy or hydrotherapy are probably the most likely treatments. Heat treatments, wax baths and electrical stimulation are all physiotherapy treatments which can relieve pain in specific joints. Hydrotherapy can be helpful for painful hip joints.

HEADACHES AND MIGRAINES

Many people worry that a headache could be caused by a brain tumour, but this is highly unlikely. The longer you have been having headaches, the less likely it is that there is a serious cause. High blood pressure rarely causes headaches. Vascular headaches are the result of stretching of the membranes around the brain, and swelling of the blood vessels within the head and neck. Tension headaches are caused by muscle tension in the neck, shoulders, scalp and face. Morning-after headaches (hangovers) are the result of drinking excessive alcohol. Migraine results in severe headache, often on one side of the head, accompanied by symptoms such as nausea, vomiting and sensory, motor and visual disturbances.

Risk: 90 per cent of people suffer at least one serious headache per year. One in four men will have a headache requiring painkillers at least once a fortnight. Only about thirty people per 100,000 per year are afflicted by brain tumours.

Recognition: we all know what a headache feels like. Doctors look for neck stiffness, very high blood pressure, pressure changes at the back of the eye, evidence that bright light hurts the sufferer and irregularity in the pupils – all these could be signs of a serious underlying cause.

Talk to your doctor if a headache worsens in the morning, wakes you during the night and came on suddenly or severely. If you notice a friend, or member of your family starting to complain of headaches, while also showing changes in personality, ask a doctor to check them over, as this might suggest a brain tumour.

Plan A: self-help prevention strategies

- If tension headaches are a problem, take up one of the relaxation techniques (see Appendix).
- Tension headaches can be caused by working hunched over a badly lit computer, in poorly ventilated surroundings. If you have any control over your office surroundings, try to ensure lighting is bright, but not harsh, and preferably not from fluorescent strips, which can cause problems for migraine sufferers. Open a window, if you can. Ask for a chair with adequate back support, and check you are comfortable with the height of your desk and keyboard.
- If you think eye strain is contributing to your problem, have your eyes tested.
- Drink plenty of water at regular intervals through the day, as fluid loss can contribute to headaches.
- Cut down on known trigger foods, such as coffee, chocolate and cheese. Avoid vitamin A.

Plan B: treatment

If you suffer from migraine, your doctor will probably prescribe a painkiller combined with an anti-sickness drug. For everyday headaches, try to resist the temptation to rely on over-the-counter painkillers, as in some circumstances these can reduce the body's ability to make natural painkillers, called endorphins, and so contribute to the headaches for which you take them.

Complementary therapies have much to offer the headache sufferer, assuming a serious underlying cause has been ruled out by your GP. Acupuncture is excellent for pain relief, and the World Health Organization recommends its use for migraine.

COMMON SKIN PROBLEMS

Skin problems are rarely dangerous, but their psychological effects can be devastating. If you are a victim, remember that unblemished skin is rarely attainable – the purpose of skin is to protect the body from dangers inherent in the environment (water, heat, cold, infection, friction, ultraviolet light, etc.). With these pressures, it is inevitable that skin breaks down from time to time. As we age, our skin thins, becomes wrinkled, and spotted with minor coloured lesions and moles.

Risk: acne is extremely common. It afflicts 6 per cent of adults throughout their lives. About 1.5 per cent of adults suffer from eczema throughout their lives. Similarly, 2 per cent of white people suffer psoriasis – it is less common in other ethnic groups. Most people suffer dermatitis – patches of dry, itchy skin, at some time. Fungal infections of the skin, such as athlete's foot, are also fairly common.

Recognition: in acne, the skin is greasy, and there are many blackheads. Eczema in adults leads to patches of red, flaky skin. In psoriasis the skin is flaky, and sheds scales very easily. Most sportsmen know all about athlete's foot – it causes intense itchiness between the toes, and the skin often cracks.

If in doubt about the diagnosis, your doctor will look at your skin through a magnifying glass, and may scrape off a tiny amount from the afflicted area, for further analysis.

Ask your doctor about any changes in the appearance of your skin which worry you – you are not wasting his or her time. Also, report any changes in the size or texture of moles, or the growth of new ones.

Plan A: self-help prevention strategies

● Examine your diet, as making changes could have a significant impact on the problem. For instance, some eczema sufferers are helped by eliminating dairy products or eggs.

● If you suffer from acne, avoid using greasy hair preparations which will clog up the pores on your forehead.

● If you suffer eczema, or dermatitis, try to ensure your skin does not dry out between flare-ups, by using any simple moisturizer.

● Psoriasis can be triggered by stress, so learn a relaxation technique (see Appendix).

- Many skin conditions can be helped by modest exposure to sunlight – although not to the point of burning.

Plan B: treatment

Eczema is mainly treated with moisturizing creams, or steroid creams, if severe. Psoriasis is treated with a variety of creams. Acne and psoriasis are both sometimes treated with ultraviolet light. Over-the-counter preparations are commonly available for athlete's foot.

Evening primrose oil helps many skin problems. It is available in creams, which can be rubbed on to the affected area (not acne), or your GP or dermatologist may be willing to prescribe it in oral form.

Under the knife – common male operations

Age brings not only wisdom but knee pains, varicose veins, prostate trouble and a host of other ailments. Here are some of the most common operations men are likely to face.

CIRCUMCISION

WHY IS IT DONE?

A common reason is religious requirements, particularly among Muslim or Jewish people. In America circumcision is recommended as a hygiene measure. The usual medical reason is phimosis, where the foreskin is scarred by recurrent infections, the tip becomes narrow, the foreskin cannot be retracted and urine sprays out. Though most common in boys, phimosis is not unusual in adult men. Cancer of the penis, admittedly unusual anyway, virtually never occurs in circumcised men.

HOW IS IT DONE?

The surgeon cuts around the foreskin close to where it joins the penis, tying off blood vessels on the way. Jewish boys are circumcised at eight days without anaesthetic by a specially trained religious surgeon.

AFTERWARDS
Whether in adults or children it takes about a week for the skin to heal. The procedure is painful for adults afterwards, but babies seem not to have any discomfort after a few hours. Complications, usually minor, include infection or persistent bleeding. Rarely the tip of the penis is damaged.

HERNIA REPAIR
WHY IS IT DONE?
A hernia is a tissue or an organ that protrudes through its surrounding tissue or muscle. Many babies are born with small hernias in the groin. Physically demanding jobs that strain the tissues in the groin often cause a hernia that gradually enlarges and becomes painful. Hernias should always be repaired to avoid the risk of strangulation, where some bowel is trapped inside the hernia.

HOW IS IT DONE?
In the traditional operation, the skin and muscle over the hernia is cut open, and repaired layer by layer either with stitches or with an artificial mesh. Increasingly repairs are done laparoscopically, through a thin tube inserted through a small cut in the groin. The repair is done from under the skin; this is a more technically demanding procedure. Hernia repair can be done under local anaesthetic.

AFTERWARDS
Babies recover within a day or two. It takes about seven to ten days to recover from classical surgery but just a day or two from keyhole surgery. Full strength takes six to twelve weeks depending on the type of repair done. Complications include persistent pain or failure of the repair.

VASECTOMY
This popular method of contraception is described on page 112.

PILES (HAEMORRHOIDS)

WHAT ARE THESE?

To those not in the medical profession, piles are best thought of as varicose veins around the back passage. Our Western low-fibre diet probably encourages piles by making it a strain to open the bowels. Piles itch, protrude and bleed.

HOW ARE THEY TREATED?

Piles only need treating if you want it. The choice is wide – injection, freezing or having tight bands placed over them. These all destroy the blood supply so the pile shrinks over a few weeks. Unfortunately piles tend to recur after a few years. Then they can be surgically cut out together with a segment of skin from the anus (in an operation called a haemorrhoidectomy).

AFTERWARDS

Banding, freezing or injection are outpatient procedures; apart from some aching you will feel fine immediately. Haemorrhoidectomy is quite a procedure; it takes two weeks at least to recover from it. You can reduce the chances of piles recurring by eating a high-fibre diet to avoid constipation.

VARICOSE VEINS

WHAT ARE THEY?

Men think only women get varicose (enlarged and twisted) veins. This is not so, though it is true that women are more prone. They occur anywhere along the legs, especially in people who spend time on their feet. Most varicose veins are just unsightly; but they may itch, become inflamed (phlebitis) or lead to ulceration of surrounding skin. Bleeding from a varicose vein is rare.

HOW ARE THEY TREATED?

To treat small individual veins a surgeon injects fluid that makes the blood inside clot, so destroying that vein. Another technique, under anaesthetic, is to cut down to the vein and tie it. Several veins can be dealt with at once. Really bad veins all down the leg are treated by stripping out the whole vein; this is a rather brutal procedure, not so often done as in later life the vein may be useful for heart surgery.

AFTERWARDS
It takes two to three weeks to recover from having a vein stripped, just a day or two for other procedures. You have to wear bandages for two to three weeks.

ARTHROSCOPY
WHY IS IT DONE?
This means looking inside a joint. It is done to investigate pain in the knee, shoulder, hip or ankle, where a specialist thinks there may be fragments of bone, a torn cartilage or ligament, or rough areas of bone. Or it is to take a biopsy of the joint to establish a diagnosis. It is often necessary after sports injuries or if a torn cartilage is suspected.

HOW IS IT DONE?
A 1cm cut by the joint is all that is needed to let the instrument inside the joint. Under its bright light the surgeon inspects the bones and cartilages, removing damaged areas, grinding down rough areas, repairing torn ligaments and biopsying bone, cartilage or the lining of the joint. Arthroscopy is usually done under general anaesthetic and takes between thirty minutes and one hour.

AFTERWARDS
You are left with one or two cuts and stitches. For most procedures you can walk almost immediately, though longer is required after a ligament repair. Pain is minimal and goes within a couple of days.

GALL BLADDER REMOVAL
WHY IS IT DONE?
The pain from gallstones is severe and likely to recur at the least convenient times, like when you are on holiday.

HOW IS IT DONE?
The preferred method of removal is by keyhole surgery, called laparoscopic cholecystectomy. Thin operating instruments are inserted via three 1cm cuts in the upper abdomen. The gall bladder lies under the liver on the upper right side of the abdomen and can normally be cut away in an operation lasting an hour or so.

If there are complications such as heavy bleeding or unusual anatomy, an open operation is required. An 8cm cut below the right ribs allows exposure of the whole operating area. Until a few years ago this was the standard gall bladder operation.

AFTERWARDS

After laparoscopic cholecystectomy you stay in hospital for only one or two days and full recovery takes two to four weeks. A seven-day stay is needed after open surgery and six to eight weeks in all to recover.

CORONARY ARTERY BYPASS GRAFTING
WHY IS IT DONE?

This is surgery to replace arteries around the heart that have become narrowed with atheroma, e.g. after investigation for angina or after a heart attack. With restored blood flow the heart can work again to its maximum efficiency and without pain.

HOW?

This is open-heart surgery; the surgeon cuts through the breastbone and levers it apart to expose the heart. Then the heart is stopped while the grafts are inserted. During this period your blood is pumped artificially through your lungs and round your body by a heart/lung machine. The graft is preferably taken from yourself – either a section of vein from the leg or artery to the breast – but artificial grafts are available. Once the grafts are in place the heart is restarted.

AFTERWARDS

You will be in intensive care for twenty-four to forty-eight hours then on a general ward. There will be stitches in the breast bone and in your leg from where the vein graft was taken. After a week you can go home, while full recovery takes eight to twelve weeks. You will have regular check-ups for a year or two afterwards.

CYSTOSCOPY AND PROSTATE SURGERY
WHY IS IT DONE?

Many men develop urinary problems by their sixties or have an enlarged prostate gland with difficulty passing urine, a need to go frequently or to go urgently. Cystoscopy may be a necessary investigation of possible cancer of the prostate or of blood in the urine.

HOW IS IT DONE?

The cystoscope is a thin metal tube passed under anaesthetic up the penis into the bladder, allowing the surgeon to inspect the walls as it passes, sampling anything that looks suspicious. If prostatectomy is required, it can be done by burning away the prostate gland with a heated wire or with a laser, all under direct vision. Cystoscopy can be done under local anaesthetic.

AFTERWARDS

Pain and discomfort lasts for two to five days as inflammation settles down. After prostatectomy you may get dribbling of urine and sperm may not be ejaculated but instead pass into the bladder (retrograde ejaculation), emerging later in the urine. Some men become impotent after extensive prostate surgery for cancer.

HIP REPLACEMENT

WHY IS IT DONE?

Osteoarthritis (wear and tear of the hip joint) causes pain, stiffness and difficulty walking. Many men who are otherwise well find this a great restriction on their activities. Emergency hip replacement is done if you fracture your hip.

HOW IS IT DONE?

A 10cm cut is made along the upper outer part of the thigh to expose the head of the thigh bone. The diseased bone (the head of the femur) is cut away, after which an artificial hip is inserted. Artifical hips are mostly metal and are secured into the thigh bone by screwing or cementing in place. If necessary an artificial cup is inserted into the pelvic bone.

AFTERWARDS

You will be helped to walk a few hours after surgery, to reduce the risk of a blood clot in the leg. You will be quite mobile after two weeks and should be fully mobile after eight to ten weeks. Hip replacement improves things for about 95 per cent of people. Artificial hips may need replacing after ten to fifteen years.

Mysterious symptoms

During the last fifty or so years, a number of diseases and disorders have emerged that seem to resist all modern medicine can throw at them, and which many doctors treat with scepticism. Here are some suggestions for minimizing your risk, and coping in a crisis.

IRRITABLE BOWEL SYNDROME

IBS is not a positive diagnosis, but what is left when other serious bowel disorders have been ruled out. There is no agreement about the cause, other than that it is something to do with the muscular wall of the bowel.

Risk: at least 40 per cent of people suffer frequent, mild abdominal pain; about 20 per cent suffer from IBS.

Recognition: there is recurrent abdominal pain, together with a feeling of distension, or bloating. The bowels may swing between constipation and diarrhoea. The symptoms can go on for months or years, yet general health is good and there is no weight loss. Doctors may investigate these symptoms via blood tests, analysis of your urine and motions, and a barium enema.

Plan A: self-help and prevention

- Examine your diet. Make sure you are getting enough fibre, by eating plenty of fruit and vegetables. Drink plenty of water each day.
- Try to avoid cigarettes, coffee and alcohol.
- Stress can be a trigger; take up one of the relaxation techniques (see Appendix).
- Keep up a regular exercise programme.

Plan B: treatment

Your GP might offer anti-spasmodic drugs, to relax the muscles of the bowel, or drugs to counteract diarrhoea. If stress is an important factor, he or she might consider prescribing a low dose of an antidepressant. Most complementary practitioners will be able to suggest ways of tackling IBS.

FOOD ALLERGY AND INTOLERANCE

Substances which are harmful to the body are dealt with by the immune system, which produces antibodies against them. In an allergic reaction to food, the immune system is over-sensitive, and treats normally harmless substances as if they were foreign invaders. It is not clear whether the immune system is involved in food intolerance, and this simply means any adverse reaction to a food.

Risk: nutritional therapists think that approximately 20 per cent of people suffer some form of food allergy, or intolerance. Allergies to shellfish, milk and nuts are common. If you suffer from asthma, eczema or hay fever you have an increased chance of suffering food allergy or intolerance. Stress is often a trigger.

Recognition: symptoms vary through a range of niggling health problems to collapse. Rashes are common. Mood swings, irritability, insomnia and anxiety have all been attributed to food allergy or intolerance, as have respiratory and digestive upsets, headaches and migraine, joint pain and more. The standard hospital test for allergies involves introducing a tiny amount of the suspect substance under the skin, and waiting to see if there is any kind of reaction. Complementary therapists may suggest hair analysis to identify allergy. GPs tend to be wary of the idea of food intolerance, but it is a standard diagnosis for nutritional therapists and naturopaths, who would probably identify the cause via an elimination diet.

Plan A: self-help and prevention

- Keep a diary of everything you eat, and everything you do, over two weeks. This may help reveal a link between a reaction, and a specific food or drink. Or it might show that dog hair, soap or your aftershave is the cause of your intolerance.
- In general, elimination diets should only be undertaken under professional guidance, but it should be safe to undertake a small-scale diet, eliminating just one food, on your own. If you suspect a specific food is causing the problem, cut it out for two weeks, but otherwise eat normally. If matters improve, you have probably identified the culprit.
- If stress triggers your reactions, explore the various relaxation techniques (see Appendix).

Plan B: treatment

Your GP might prescribe antihistamine drugs to control symptoms produced by an allergy. Most complementary therapists will be able to suggest ways of treating specific symptoms of allergy, or intolerance. For example, there are homoeopathic remedies for headaches or rashes – and a registered homoeopath might also have some success in developing a desensitizing programme.

ANDROPAUSE (MALE MENOPAUSE)

Unlike the clearly defined female menopause, the whole concept of andropause, the male menopause, is controversial. Nevertheless, increasing numbers of men are reporting puzzling symptoms which appear when they are about forty-five and disappear by sixty-five. More research is needed, but scientists are beginning to take seriously the possibility that these symptoms could be due to less efficient production of the male hormone testosterone.

Risk: if andropause is a genuine phenomenon, then all men will go through it, in the same way that all women go through the menopause.

Recognition: reported symptoms include dizziness, tiredness, low energy levels, impotence and declining libido, night sweats, irritability, mood swings, headaches, joint pain and digestive upsets.

Plan A: self-help and prevention

Women cannot prevent the menopause, and neither, if it is real, can you prevent the andropause. However, there are a number of steps you can take to ease your transition from youth, through mid-life, to older age.

- Eat small amounts regularly, rather than big meals with large gaps between them. This will guard against swings in your blood sugar level – these aggravate many symptoms. Eat plenty of fresh fruit and vegetables, but avoid sugar and sweet foods, fatty foods and refined white flour – all can play havoc with blood-sugar levels.
- Avoid alcohol and caffeine, which can aggravate symptoms. Replace coffee and tea with herbal teas, fruit juices, or water.
- Make sure you are getting regular exercise, but not jogging, or anything else that could cause jarring, as your joints are not as

robust as those of a younger man. Cycling and brisk walking are excellent forms of exercise.

- Relaxation techniques can be an invaluable tool for easing stress at this time – see Appendix for suggestions.

Plan B: treatment

If you are persistent and manage to persuade your GP to accept the notion of the andropause, you may be lucky enough to be placed on testosterone replacement therapy. However, this is not widely available on the NHS, and you may find you have to pay for treatment at specialist clinics.

Complementary practitioners are likely to be more willing to accept the notion of andropause. Western herbalism offers herbs to reduce the severity of a range of problems – borage helps to support the adrenal glands, taking the strain off your hormonal system, for example. Evening primrose oil helps regulate body processes.

ME/CFS

ME (myalgic encephalomyelitis), or CFS (chronic fatigue syndrome), is a condition of severe chronic tiredness. Debility after a viral infection, such as glandular fever, is common. To qualify for a diagnosis of CFS, you must show symptoms for at least six months.

Risk: reliable statistics are not available, but one Australian study suggests that just over twelve males per 100,000 suffer from CFS. Young adults are most at risk, and most sufferers are from the higher social classes. There is a high incidence of depression and anxiety in sufferers.

Recognition: persistent, debilitating tiredness is the major symptom. Other symptoms include mental confusion, or difficulty in concentrating, over-sensitivity to touch and allergens, insomnia, mood swings, muscle aches, abdominal pains and reduced ability to fight minor infections, such as thrush. There are no formal diagnostic investigations carrying scientific validity.

Plan A: self-help and prevention

- Diet – eat a well-balanced diet, with plenty of wholefoods.
- Exertion within the limits of your ability will help overcome debility. If you can manage it, try to go for a short walk each day.

Tai chi is a gentle form of exercise which could offer you significant benefits.
- The stresses of living with CFS can be counteracted by many relaxation techniques (see page 148 for suggestions).

Plan B: treatment

Your GP may suggest a low dose of an antidepressant. Complementary therapists offer a range of treatments, but always discuss these with your GP. Do not attempt self-treatment, as you are likely to be sensitive to medication of any sort, including natural medicines.

TAT (TIRED ALL THE TIME)

This is a recently described syndrome which seems to be a response to the demands of a modern, highly technological lifestyle – little privacy, and less time to ourselves. It is not as debilitating as CFS.

Risk: in one survey, 25 per cent of people selected at random reported they felt constantly fatigued. Both sexes were affected equally.

Recognition: the symptoms are constant tiredness, and insomnia caused by worry.

Plan A: self-help and prevention

There are a number of measures you can take to help prevent insomnia and TAT. See page 35 for suggested action for sleep problems.

SAD (SEASONAL AFFECTIVE DISORDER)

SAD is linked to light deficiency. Light stops the body producing melatonin, a sleep hormone. Lack of light allows uninhibited production of melatonin, which plays havoc with the body clock, while simultaneously suppressing production of seratonin, a chemical which carries messages in the brain and whose lack slows the body down. If you suffer from SAD you will become severely depressed in winter, when the days are short, sunlight is watery, and cloud cover tends to be dense. You may become wildly elated in spring as the days start to lengthen.

Risk: Just under 20 per cent of the population is estimated to suffer from some form of SAD; of these about 3 per cent are very severely incapacitated in winter. Women are more likely to come forward than men, but it is probable that men and women are equally affected. There may be a genetic risk of suffering SAD, although nothing is proven.

Recognition: as the days start to shorten, you will start to feel gloomy, sad and worried, your moods will get blacker as winter progresses. You may sleep badly, and stop eating. Physical symptoms might include headache and backache, panic attacks and loss of libido. Your behaviour may become irrational. As the days start to lengthen all these symptoms begin to improve. A minority of sufferers experience extreme elation (mania) in spring.

Plan A: self-help and prevention

Maximize the amount of light you receive by sleeping with the curtains open, working by a window, if possible, and taking regular walks during daylight hours. Even if the weather is cold, try to expose your face, and if possible, your arms, to the light. If you can afford to, take a winter holiday, and travel to somewhere with intense light, such as the Caribbean.

Plan B: treatment

Your GP might prescribe an antidepressant, such as Prozac. Otherwise you can try light treatment. Light boxes are available, which simulate natural daylight. Depending on the severity of your symptoms, you may need to sit in front of your box for between half an hour and four hours per day. Contact the SAD Association if you require further information (see Useful Addresses).

SBS (SICK BUILDING SYNDROME)

Sick building syndrome refers to a group of symptoms which can all be attributed to working in high-tech, air-conditioned and centrally heated offices. Symptoms include constantly itchy eyes, and an endlessly runny nose, a persistent cough, headaches, tiredness and general aches and pains.

Risk: no statistics are available, but if you work in a high-rise building, where the windows are sealed shut and all air is recycled through a central unit, where most light is artificial and there is constant background noise – from the hum of computers, as well as human chatter – you could be at risk.

Recognition: do you have unexplained symptoms of the type listed above? If so, and there is no other explanation, and you are otherwise in good health, it might be that your working environment is to blame. No formal diagnostic investigations are possible.

Plan A: self-help and prevention

Perhaps feng shui provides your greatest hope of avoiding SBS. This is the ancient Chinese system of arranging our environment so that we can live in harmony with our surroundings – the idea is to allow chi (energy) to flow slowly around things, not to be forced to shoot down rigid pathways. Could you persuade your company to seek the advice of a consultant? If not, try to ensure your desk is placed diagonally across the corner of your office, and that you face the door. If you share an office, or work in an open-plan environment, try to ensure that desks are not arranged in straight lines. Long corridors should be broken-up as far as possible, even introducing a bank of filing cabinets into a corridor could help. Doors should not face each other across corridors, but should be slightly offset. Plants are very useful for breaking up sharp chi, and cheer up even the most soulless office.

Plan B: treatment

Your GP may be willing to prescribe drugs to deal with your individual symptoms. Most complementary therapists could also offer remedies to counteract the worst effects of SBS. Crystal therapy could help – rose quartz absorbs harmful radiation from computers, and amethyst is the source of healing vibrations.

ADD (ATTENTION DEFICIT DISORDER)

This disorder is characterized by a lack of ability to concentrate or focus on an activity or project for more than a few moments at a time.

Risk: very few figures are available. Most studies have been done on children, not adults. They show that boys are four times more likely to suffer than girls.

Recognition: in addition to inability to concentrate, other symptoms include irritability, hyperactivity and restlessness, insomnia, mood swings and sometimes anti-social behaviour and violence. You probably will not recognize these symptoms in yourself, but your friends, colleagues and family members may force you to confront them.

Plan A: self-help and prevention

- Examine your diet. Highly processed foods containing additives and colorants have been implicated in the condition. Try to eat fresh, wholefoods, especially fruit and vegetables.
- Make sure you are getting plenty of exercise.
- Take up one of the relaxation techniques suggested on page 148. The breathing exercise described there and meditation both offer demanding work-outs for your powers of concentration.
- To ensure a good night's sleep, see page 35 and TAT above.

Plan B: treatment

Aggression control classes could help – they show you how to recognize and defuse aggression. Arts therapies could also provide support. These aim to alleviate emotional problems by encouraging you to express and understand feelings through an arts medium, such as music, movement, drama, painting or modelling in clay.

Hangovers – and what to do about them

So, you were out on a bender with the guys last night? Got drunk, went for a curry, drank some more, and finally collapsed into a cab, just managing to mumble your address before passing out? Now your partner refuses to speak to you, instead she's throwing you 'you'll get no sympathy from me' looks. Your mouth feels like the bottom of a parrot's cage, your head is throbbing, your guts seem to be about to explode and you can't hold your hands steady. What can you do?

- If you have a raging thirst and your head throbs in direct proportion to the number of drinks you downed last night, you are dehydrated. Drink at least two pints of water. Continue to drink water through the day. Do not eat until the hangover has passed.
- Force yourself to get out of bed, or off the sofa, and go for a walk in the fresh air. Exercise gets the blood pumping, supplying

oxygen and sugar to the brain, while stimulating the release of natural painkillers (endorphins).

- Once you are home, settle down in front of the TV or a mindless video – and remind yourself that recovery from a hangover is normally just a matter of time.
- Bach Rescue Remedy (available from health-food shops and pharmacies) is a handy stand-by to counteract some of the psychological aspects of hangover – remorse, depression and general unhappiness.
- Nux vomica is a homoeopathic remedy suitable for headaches accompanied by nausea and irritability following over-indulgence of food, coffee and alcohol. It will help banish any heavy feelings at the base of your skull, and will reduce over-sensitivity to noise.
- Herbal teas made from camomile, peppermint, ginger or thyme will help settle your stomach.
- Apologize profusely to your partner.

Now here is a quick lesson in why over-indulgence produces the typical symptoms of hangover. Alcohol is toxic to the brain – probably because it interferes with the transmission of nerve impulses from brain cell to brain cell, thus playing havoc with our higher functions. This initially has an anaesthetic effect, which is why our sense of inhibition and sensitivity to others' reactions are reduced when we drink.

Alcohol is a potent dilator of blood vessels – so drinkers look flushed. The headache in a hangover is caused by dilation of blood vessels in the scalp and around the brain. A headache persisting after most of the alcohol has left the body is thought to be caused by breakdown products, or factors such as smoking, loss of sleep or dehydration.

As well as irritating the stomach lining, alcohol also has a diuretic effect – it causes the kidneys to pass out more fluid than the volume drunk. This is why hangover is often accompanied by thirst.

Alcoholic drinks are not pure alcohol; they contain a variety of other substances, called congeners, which give them their character. These congeners are believed to be even more toxic than pure alcohol, and give rise to many of the symptoms of hangover, such as shakiness, vertigo and nausea. Congeners are in highest concentration in drinks such as port and brandy, and in lowest concentration in purer spirits such as gin and vodka.

Many suggestions have been made for the prevention of hangover, but only reduced consumption of alcohol will offer genuine help. If you regularly overindulge, see page 33 for advice on quitting alcohol.

Programme for change

Part One of this book has been about getting the most from your body, preventing possible health problems, and increasing your levels of strength and stamina to improve your life now and in the future. Whatever your starting point, everyone can benefit from higher levels of fitness, and greater body-awareness. Use this programme for change as a first step to a new you.

Step 1: identify what you want to change

Are you most concerned about changing your diet, getting fit, quitting smoking, cutting down on alcohol, reducing your chance of dying from heart disease or cancer, making changes in how you cope with a long-term, chronic health problem...or what?

Only you can decide what you want to change. Start by drawing up a wish list of six targets for change. Let's take Pete as an example. Pete is in his late thirties, married with two children, and has a highly stressful job as a marketing director for an international pharmaceuticals company. He describes his fitness level as 'above average, but not spectacular'. He is a member of a gym and works out 'fairly regularly'. In his teens he suffered a rugby injury which has left him with nagging back pains; he has tried various methods of dealing with this problem, but none have succeeded. He feels that the poor design of his work-station contributes to his problem.

Pete's list of targets for change are: do something about my back pain; learn about stress-control; increase my stamina; spend at least thirty minutes three times a week on cardiovascular exercise; cut down on caffeine, especially in the evening; get eight hours' sleep each night.

Step 2: set your priorities

You are unlikely to be able to tackle six targets all at once. Think about your wish list for a few days, and whittle it down to a short list of three. Pete's short list read: do something about my back; spend at least thirty minutes three times a week on cardiovascular exercise; cut down on caffeine at night.

Consider your short list for a further few days – you are not in a race to change your life. Then choose one target, one area you would like to change, which you feel would have the greatest impact on your health. Once you have achieved change in this key area, and reaped the benefits, you can come back to your other short-list choices. Pete's biggest priority for improving his physical health is to do something about his recurrent back pain.

Step 3: identify potential obstacles

If you identify potential problems in advance, you can think about how to overcome them and are less likely to be derailed by them.

The main obstacle preventing Pete from tackling his back pain is that he does not know its cause. Also, he has become dispirited by the failure of the various methods of pain control he has tried. He is unwilling to rely on painkillers. He thinks his company would be unresponsive to requests to redesign his work-station.

How could Pete overcome these obstacles? After discussion with his wife, and with his GP, Pete decided to consult a chiropractor, to see if he or she could identify the cause of the problem. If the cause could be established, then there might be hope of relief. Pete had not tried chiropractic before, and felt 'reasonably hopeful – although not too optimistic'.

He also resolved to talk to his personnel department to see if they would at least invest in a new office chair which would offer full support to his back (he met an immediately sympathetic response and had a new chair within a fortnight).

Step 4: set a timetable

How long are you prepared to give yourself before you expect to see results? Your timetable will, of course, depend on your individual aim – you cannot lose two stone in two weeks, you cannot get fitter overnight – but you must have some sense of time pressure, otherwise your project is likely to drift. Pete decided to give Dominic, his chiropractor, a total of six sessions in which to make an impact. After this Pete felt the costs of chiropractic treatment would start to be prohibitive, and that he would lose motivation to attend.

Step 5: review progress

In order to review progress, we suggest you keep a health diary specifically for this purpose. Jot down anything which seems relevant to your chosen aim. For example, Dominic gave Pete a whole series of brief exercises to work through at home. Two weeks into his treatment, Pete's entry read: 'I must look barmy standing up against the wall wrapped in my towel, doing strange lifts and jerks! But I can feel that the exercises are really helping. My lower back feels much looser, and I'm sure I can twist further to the side now than I could before. But my back still aches if I have to stand for long periods – I must remember to ask Dominic about this.'

If you notice that progress is becoming stalled, you will need to take immediate remedial action, to prevent the situation deteriorating. You might need to re-motivate yourself by reviewing the negative effects of old styles of behaviour, and the positive benefits you are aiming to achieve. Or you might need to get further professional advice, or to change direction entirely. If chiropractic had not worked for Pete, perhaps he could have asked his GP about referring him for surgery.

Step 6: reward achievement

If you succeed in your aims, plan to give yourself a health-related reward. Pete decided that if he could make significant improvements in the way he handled his back pain, he would take his wife away for a weekend in the country without the kids – the fresh air and time alone together would do them both good, and let them recharge their batteries.

Only you can decide what would reward your achievement, but ideas might include buying yourself a piece of exercise equipment; joining a gym, going walking or climbing with friends for a weekend; buying a new cycle helmet (or even a new bike). Let your imagination run free; if you succeed, you deserve a treat. If you fail, remember you did well to try, and you can always try again.

PART TWO
sexual
HEALTH

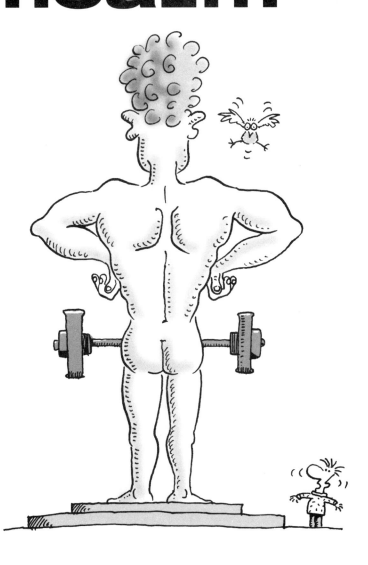

The basics of sex

SEXUAL ANATOMY

What happens during sex? What does arousal mean and what happens during intercourse?

Men's sexually responsive areas are the penis, testicles and to a lesser extent the nipples. In women they are the clitoris, which is like a small penis just above the opening of the vagina, the lips of the vagina itself and the nipples. What these regions share is erectile tissue – a structure which when engorged with blood becomes firmer and larger. They are also richly endowed with nerve endings that will transmit stimulation to the central nervous system.

Many other areas and activities are sexually stimulating during a period of foreplay – the ear lobes, the mouth, behind the knees and the inner thighs, and stroking generally. Smell is thought to be especially important; not honest sweat, but secretions from special sweat glands in the armpits, around the nipples and about the genitalia. These are called apocrine glands and their secretions, called pheromones, stimulate sexual desire.

HOW SEX IS CONTROLLED

The centre of sexual arousal is in the hypothalamus, a small structure in the base of the brain that regulates many other fundamental human functions such as hunger, thirst and sleep. The hypothalamus has nerve connections to other parts of the brain involved in pleasure, fear and pain.

The hypothalamus sends nerve messages to centres in the spinal cord that control erection in the lowest parts of the spinal cord, known as the sacral erection centre, and another known as the sympathetic thoraco-lumbar centre. These centres can and are influenced by more conscious brain messages, telling your body in effect to get on with it or to cut it out.

In women the nerve pathways are less well understood but believed to be approximately the same as in men.

PREPARING FOR SEX

The process of sexual arousal starts almost anywhere but in the genital region; it will be a thought, a look, a promise, a touch. It is helped by a loving and trusting relationship, relaxed comfortable surroundings and should be enhanced by the memory of previously pleasurable lovemaking. It will be further stimulated by a certain atmosphere – perhaps the smell of another person, music, or food. All this adds up to anticipation. Your conscious mind recognizes this with a growing sense of expectation. Actually your conscious mind may well have planned the whole situation. At an unconscious level your hypothalamus goes on alert, and then begins to transmit the nerve messages that prepare your body for sex.

FOREPLAY

Foreplay is not just a matter of being polite. Is an essential part of sex, more so for women than men, as women normally take longer to become sexually prepared than men. While a man can be fully erect within a few seconds it is likely to take a woman several minutes to reach a similar stage of readiness. Foreplay includes touching, licking and stroking the sexually sensitive areas to build up excitement. Foreplay also involves looking at each other, kissing, murmuring endearments and even giggling at getting a foot stuck in the bedclothes. Gradually the woman's lubrication begins, the muscles around the vagina relax and the time approaches for further stimulation towards intercourse and orgasm.

AROUSAL AND ORGASM IN MEN

Men reach arousal rapidly; in fact they need no mental input at all because arousal can occur through a pure spinal reflex from those centres mentioned above. This is what happens during wet dreams and the reflex erection of a baby's penis when his nappy is changed.

Under the control of nerve impulses, the blood flow in the penis changes to let more blood enter through its arteries and less escape through its veins. Tissues rich in blood vessels along the shaft of the penis fill with blood – making the penis lengthen, thicken and become erect. By a similar process the testicles also increase in size by about a third. The whole penis becomes extra sensitive to stroking or gripping, especially the tip. This is important because the penis will be gripped by the engorged walls of the vagina during intercourse, adding to the pleasure of the activity.

With increasing sexual excitement, the man's body prepares for ejaculation. Glands at the base of the penis, the bulbo-urethral glands, release a lubricant substance that leaks out of the tip of the penis. Even deeper glands, the seminal vesicles and the prostate gland provide secretions which activate sperm and which in fact make up the bulk of the ejaculate; this is called seminal fluid. Muscular contractions in these structures now secrete the fluids and move sperm along ready to be ejaculated.

Ejaculation occurs in two stages; sperm firstly has to gather at the back of the urethra which is near the root of the penis. The presence of sperm stimulates the strong muscular contractions that force out the sperm and the seminal fluid. Both processes are still under higher brain control but only up to a certain point of no return.

With the psychological experience of orgasm there is a series of urgent contractions in muscles at the base of the penis causing ejaculation. The contractions occur five to ten times over a few seconds, emitting 2–5ml of semen, after which the penis rapidly loses its erection as blood once again flows from the veins.

AROUSAL IN WOMEN

As a result of sexual excitement the hypothalamus in the brain sends its messages down through the spinal cord, in turn influencing the erectile tissues of the nipples, clitoris and the lips of the vagina. As blood pours into these structures they enlarge. At the same time secretions ooze from the walls of the vagina, moistening it and which will make intercourse more comfortable. The vagina elongates and balloons in size internally, allowing more comfortable insertion of the penis. This process takes a few minutes and will be helped by stimulation of the clitoris by finger or tongue.

Once the penis is inside the vagina, its movements may continue to stimulate the clitoris, the extent varying from woman to woman. With that continuing stimulation of the clitoris a women may reach an orgasm. At this moment she experiences rapid waves of intense sensation spreading from the clitoris across the inner thighs and the mental stimulation of a peak of sexual excitement. Internally there are waves of contractions of the vagina, the fallopian tubes and the womb, presumably to aid the passage of sperm to the egg.

AFTER ORGASM

It takes a man some time before he can be aroused again and have another orgasm; how long depends on age. Young men could be ready again within fifteen minutes whereas an elderly man may not achieve arousal for twenty-four hours. Women by contrast after a brief resting period are usually capable of another orgasm.

THE ACT OF INTERCOURSE

Above are the mechanics; there is much more to intercourse than that. This is the difference between making love or having sex. In making love the whole of each partner's body is involved – the stroking and rubbing all adding to the sexual excitement. There may be moments when the woman guides her partner to the most pleasurable actions for her and times when the man is pleasured by his partner.

The various positions for intercourse (see Injecting some spice, page 121) assist one or other to have greater excitement, often by allowing one partner to rub or stimulate the other's penis or clitoris during intercourse.

Some myths about sex

THE GOAL OF SEX IS INTERCOURSE

Intercourse is more important to men than women, who can achieve orgasm without penetration through stroking and manipulation. One of the methods of dealing with impotence in men is to ban intercourse and concentrate instead on mutual stimulation (see below).

MEN ARE ALWAYS READY

This is usually true, but many men are affected by worry, alcohol or organic illness and may even therefore resent their partner taking the initiative.

SUCCESSFUL SEX MEANS SIMULTANEOUS ORGASM

This is one of the hoariest myths of all. Surveys (don't even ask...) suggest that a third of women can reach orgasm simultaneously thanks to the movement of the penis, some of those having multiple orgasms. Many others need continuing direct stimulation of the clitoris to achieve an orgasm quite apart from the movement of the penis, and may well not have an orgasm at all in each and every act of intercourse.

SEX ENDS AT FORTY

As it gets increasingly acceptable for older people to talk about their sexual desires, it is clear that the sex remains important through the menopause and well into old age. Though women tend to lose interest more than men, men stay sexually active well into their seventies and beyond and can still father children well into old age. Nor does sexual desire necessarily wane as you get older. Some women report that their sexual appetite increases after the menopause.

Gay sexual relationships

Surveys suggest that between 3–5 per cent of men have experienced homosexual (gay) sex. A higher percentage – perhaps 6 per cent – experience some attraction towards other men, though often only as a temporary phase during adolescence. Certain cities have much higher percentages, through attracting practising gay men to that region. Since the 1970s there has been an increasingly open tolerance of gay relationships, with even legal processes accepting their validity – in relation to adopting children, for instance.

IS THERE A 'CAUSE'?

There are several theories of psychological causes of which the strongest is of being brought up in a family where the mother was dominant over the father. Other theories suggest a genetic component to being gay. These are hotly contested views, with no firm evidence favouring any particular theory.

HOW DO YOU KNOW IF YOU ARE GAY?

It is normal to experience an attraction towards other boys (or men) during adolescence, as part of the process of determining your own personality and learning to cope with emergent sexual feelings. In certain all-male environments, like boarding schools and when playing sport, such feelings may progress to physical sexual experiences. This does not make you gay but simply experimenting and many young adults will go on to have sexual relationships exclusively with women. Those who are truly gay find that sexual contact with men is far preferable to sexual contact with women; they may well find the thought of heterosexual intercourse positively repulsive. More often, surveys suggest that relatively few gay men are exclusively gay; most have both gay and heterosexual relationships.

Before reaching this stage, you may experience emotions of shame or guilt, reflecting a conflict between the way your emotions are pulling you and the way your upbringing is pushing you (towards male/female relationships). Nowadays, the guilt is lessened by the general tolerance of gay relationships, whereas not so long ago the disapproval of society drove gay men into furtive and dangerous deceptions.

GAY RELATIONSHIPS

Society generally now accepts that gay relationships can be every bit as deep and enduring as heterosexual ones. In addition (a big addition) being gay on the whole no longer puts an individual at some special risk of blackmail or threat or an undefined 'lack of reliability'. It is just an aspect of their personality which is usually irrelevant to how well they do their job. Exceptions still apply in some areas, such as working for children's organizations, situations where society is still sorting out its attitudes.

GAY SEX

The range of sexual contact includes mutual masturbation, oral-genital sex, anal sex and stimulation around the anus. Anal sex carries a high risk of transmission of a number of infections, the reason being that infections can penetrate through the skin of the anal region via tiny abrasions that occur during gay sex. The particular diseases are HIV/AIDS, syphilis, and hepatitis B, C and D. The risk is increased by the fact that some gay men have casual sex with many partners. AIDS in particular has cut a swathe through gay communities around the world, even though recent treatment advances can reduce the risk of developing AIDS after being infected by HIV (the virus responsible).

SAFE SEX

This means avoiding high-risk activities, such as anal sex, or using protective measures such as tough condoms. It includes knowing the HIV status of your sexual partners. Remember that the virus is also spread through intravenous drug use, so sex with a drug user is also risky. There is a chance of acquiring HIV/AIDS through heterosexual sex; though this is a relatively low risk at present, it is one thought likely to increase in significance over the next ten to twenty years.

Safe sex – who's really having it?

We are living in the age of HIV/AIDS and so we must all think about safe sex. Safe for whom? As a man you want to know that you are not picking up diseases from your sexual partner. But as a responsible man you will not want to put your partner at risk either. What is there to worry about?

HIV/AIDS

The HIV virus is not a remote risk; it is now the commonest cause of chronic ill health and death for millions of people in Africa and Asia. In the developed world, it is thought that HIV is a risk only to certain groups. This is true still, but HIV is predicted to spread into the heterosexual population over the next twenty years.

Risk

You catch HIV from another infected individual carrying it in their blood and sperm, but it has to get into your bloodstream. This can happen in various ways:

- Intravenous drug users will get it from needles shared by HIV-positive individuals.
- If you have anal sex, the extra trauma causes small tears through which the HIV virus can enter.
- Rarely you may catch it through having normal vaginal intercourse with an HIV-positive person. This is unlikely but is predicted to become common.
- If you have oral sex, infected fluids may enter through small cuts or sores in your mouth or from sores on your partner's genitalia.

Recognition

The initial infection causes a trivial viral-type illness. Once infected you will almost certainly eventually develop AIDS, but this can take ten years or more. AIDS begins with weight loss, and unusual infections (usually chest infections) but later causes widespread ill health through destruction of the immune system.

So you will not know that you have caught HIV without a blood test. This goes positive three months after infection. If you think your behaviour has been high risk, see a specialized AIDS centre for counselling or a blood test. Do not have sex with anyone until you know your HIV status.

Safe sex

As far as AIDS goes you reduce your risk by:

- wearing a condom for vaginal, anal or oral sex unless you know your partner is clear;
- not using intravenous drugs;
- not having casual sex with high risk individuals i.e. homosexuals, bisexual men, or people in high-risk countries of Asia and Africa.

SEXUALLY TRANSMITTED DISEASES

If you follow the guidelines for avoiding HIV, you are unlikely to run into problems with other sexually transmitted diseases; but here is what to look out for.

Syphilis

This was the AIDS of its time (the nineteenth century) but is now uncommon in the UK. You get it through normal intercourse or anal intercourse with someone who is infected.

RECOGNITION

- a painless sore on the penis, anus or mouth a few weeks after infection;
- enlarged glands in the armpits and groin;
- a sparse rash on the whole body including the hands and feet;
- after a few months fleshy warts around the genitalia.

Then the disease goes quiet. Years later it can reactivate causing:

- collapse of bones;
- dementia;
- sudden brief but severe shooting pains in the limbs;
- heart disease;
- transmission to unborn children, causing congenital syphilis, with bone and nervous system damage as in adults.

TREATMENT

The disease is diagnosed by swabs and blood tests. Treatment is not difficult but does involve ten days of penicillin injections.

Gonorrhoea

There is a bigger risk of catching gonorrhoea than syphilis as it is far more common in the UK.

RISK

You can get gonorrhoea from normal or anal intercourse with an infected person.

RECOGNITION

A few days after exposure you get burning when passing urine then a cloudy discharge from your penis. If you had anal intercourse you may get rectal itching. Without treatment often the disease will go. However, you should still be concerned because if you pass it on to a woman, it is highly likely to cause internal infection and chronic pelvic inflammation leading to infertility. And she may not even know she has had the disease until she finds she is infertile.

TREATMENT
This is even easier than syphilis and only involves a single high-dose of an antibiotic.

Hepatitis B
RISK
You catch this virus through anal intercourse, as it is carried in blood and sperm. The other route is through intravenous drug use.

RECOGNITION
The virus incubates for two weeks to six months; then after a brief flu-like illness you become jaundiced (yellow), often with pain over the liver. Though this clears up there is a permanent greatly increased risk of liver cancer and about a 1 per cent risk of liver failure.

TREATMENT
There is none really effective. You will pose a permanent risk of infecting others if you give blood or have an operation.

Other sexually transmitted diseases
The commonest is called NSU (non-specific urethritis); others are thrush, trichomonas, herpes and chlamydia. These are the ones found most frequently in the Western world; there are plenty of more exotic things you can get in the tropics.

RECOGNIZING SEXUALLY TRANSMITTED DISEASE
Be aware of:

● sores on the penis;
● itching around the genital region;
● discharge from the penis;
● warts around the penis or anus.

TREATMENT

Go to a clinic for sexually transmitted diseases – most towns have them and you will be treated in confidence. You will need swabs taken from your penis, anus and mouth, and blood tests to ensure you have not picked up other illnesses. Treatment for many sexually transmitted diseases is straightforward – creams or tablets, except for the blood-borne ones mentioned earlier.

Sexually transmitted illnesses are often relatively trivial for men (AIDS and hepatitis apart) but can be devastating for women. You are no one's hero if you shrug off these problems.

PREVENTION

Read again the previous sections on avoiding HIV and how to have safe sex. In brief:

- wear a condom;
- be extremely careful if having anal sex or sexual activity with a homosexual, bisexual or intravenous drug user. Do not have intercourse if you have a sore in your mouth or anus, and take seriously the symptoms of sexually transmitted disease given earlier.

Common sexual queries and problems

See also Injecting some spice, page 121.

SIZE OF PENIS – DOES IT MATTER?

If you are hung like a horse, but call a woman by the wrong name, never kiss her during sex and won't allow contact between any body parts except the actual genitalia, then no woman is likely to stick around for long... If you are worried about size, remember that however big or small your penis is when limp, when erect all men are about equal in size at 4½–6 inches in length.

Men may never quite believe these statistics – but there is no way to prove otherwise without getting arrested. As long as you are in an established and happy relationship which includes sex, you can accept that there is mutual satisfaction, whatever the physical size.

SHOULD SEX ALWAYS END IN PENETRATION?

Men who ask this tend to mean 'Will you give me a blow job?' This is up to your partner – ask her. If she is happy about oral sex, remember to return the favour, and however much you are tempted, never, ever, push her head down, even if that is the direction you want her to go. It is all about variety really – and fantasy. Often men reserve more experimental sex for an occasional partner (or prostitute) and stick to more conventional sex with their regular partner.

HOW CAN I TELL WHAT MY PARTNER ENJOYS?

If you want to learn what your partner likes, try asking her! Or allow her to show you during sex, or simply watch what she does. There are many ways a man can give a woman pleasure – make her glad she has breasts by handling them with care, kissing and caressing them; kiss her all over, massage her; use your hands or your tongue prior to penetration, and so on.

Men do realize this deep down, but it can be a problem to know how to ask, especially early on in a relationship. With women taking the initiative more in sex, perhaps these areas will become easier to navigate – and more fun.

CIRCUMCISION – WHAT'S THE WOMAN'S ATTITUDE?

Men on the whole do not go out of their way to get circumcised, unless pain and infection drives us to it. No woman wants to be faced with a dirty, smelly penis, encrusted with cheesy secretions under the foreskin. If you are not circumcised, wash regularly! In other words, circumcision doesn't matter either way to a woman, as long as you are clean.

MY PENIS APPEARS DEFORMED BY A CURVE

Many men develop a curve in later life – it is called Peyronie's disease. Not a lot can be done for minor curves. If a curve is so great that intercourse is getting difficult, see a urologist. There are operations to help – but be warned, they are rather drastic.

MY FORESKIN IS TIGHT

An adult should be able to retract his foreskin easily to wash under it and before intercourse. If you cannot do this, it may be that your foreskin has become scarred and inelastic through repeated mild infections of the foreskin called balanitis. If bad enough, you will need a circumcision – this is not at all unusual in adult men.

I DON'T WANT SEX SO MUCH ANY MORE

This is only a problem if your partner wants sex all the time, and you don't. Often it is a part of getting used to each other; though sex may have been the initial attraction, other things in a relationship become important with time. If in an established relationship both of you are happy with lower levels of sexual activity than you enjoyed when you were first together, then fine. If she wants sex far more often than you, then the two of you need to talk over your situation – see also Erection problems and I find it hard to discuss sex with my partner (below).

I CAN NEVER TELL WHEN A WOMAN WANTS SEX

Here is a clue – it probably sounds obvious! If a woman gets into bed, turns her back on you and says 'I'm going to sleep now', she does not want sex. If, on the other hand, she gets into bed and starts stroking sensitive parts of your body... If you are genuinely uncertain, try kissing her neck or shoulders, and see where that gets you. The trouble is that men get aroused so easily. Perhaps you should remember to keep a good book at hand!

HOW WOULD A WOMAN FEEL IF WE STOPPED HAVING SEX SO REGULARLY?

It depends what you think counts as regular. Once a week is regular, but so is once every six months. If sex suddenly drops off for no apparent reason, many women would be suspicious, but if you have been together a long time, and you both have many demands and responsibilities (perhaps work or children), then most women would probably accept a diminution in desire as understandable. It is worth talking this over together, remembering that depression and worry are the usual reasons why a man loses interest in sex.

Regard it as reassuring if your partner says she misses sex; this should give you confidence about the relationship and help you towards overcoming any short-term problems. There are lots of additional reasons why a man might go off sex long term (or fail to get an erection) – drinking to excess, physical problems like diabetes and poor blood flow in the lower body. Or it may be that your sex life has gone stale; read page 121 for some advice.

ERECTION PROBLEMS

Generally speaking if you get an erection on waking or at certain other times, there is unlikely to be a physical cause for erection problems. In a healthy relationship your partner will almost certainly be prepared to try the arousal techniques you find helpful. If she is not prepared to help, this might indicate fundamental difficulties between you, which could, indeed, be the cause of your erection problems – at least in part. In this case, you might benefit from professional relationship counselling. It comes down to communication again.

If, however, you consistently fail to get an erection in all circumstances, you should have a medical check to exclude factors mentioned earlier such as diabetes, poor blood flow, side-effects of medication or of alcohol, as well as more serious anxiety or depression.

Aids to impotence include Viagra, see page 104, and self-injection with a drug which causes erection. Not all men cope with this – it takes training to overcome natural fears – but it works well. You may also be able to get help for impotence in tablet form.

Another simple aid is a rubber ring placed around the base of the penis. This prevents blood leaving the penis and so keeps it erect. High technology for impotence comes in the form of inflatable rods implanted within the penis – a last resort but an effective one.

I SEEM TO REACH ORGASM VERY QUICKLY

It is no fun for women that they take longer to come than men. Your partner will understand that you get so excited you cannot help coming quickly, but she will still be fed up if you then make her feel that any further ministrations from you are fuelled by politeness, and nothing more.

Men would like to slow down too. This means taking more time over foreplay and learning what you each like; try to engage in lots of foreplay to bring your partner to orgasm, or close to it, prior to penetration. As for reaching orgasm together during intercourse – this is a really difficult issue. Even sex experts cannot agree whether this is the norm or not; their surveys suggest that relatively few couples do achieve simultaneous orgasm during intercourse. If your partnership is not one of those, it is up to the man to learn how to give his partner satisfaction before penetration.

The following techniques are well established in sex therapy. You spend time giving each other mutual pleasure but stopping short of intercourse. That means stroking, licking, and rubbing.

If you feel embarrassed about giving your partner oral sex, or about using your hand on her, think about whether you feel embarrassed about her giving you oral sex, or using her hand to bring you off. You'd probably willingly accept either of the latter; if so, it is simply not fair to refuse to use your hands or tongue on her.

And what can you do if you feel you are coming? Try the squeeze technique – ask your partner to grip your penis firmly under the tip. It will stop your orgasm in its tracks, guaranteed. Once you both know how to control orgasm, you can be more relaxed about sexual foreplay.

I FANCY SOME EXPERIMENTATION

Variety is fun, at least many men think so. You might like trying new positions, but your partner might find many of them uncomfortable. So you must each let each other know how it is for you. Ask your partner! Many women are happy to experiment. If your partner laughs, she's not into it. If she laughs in a derisive 'who the hell do you think you are?' sort of way, she's certainly not into it…

You may like to experiment with bondage and stuff, but your partner may well not be happy about that, and feel nervous about telling you. But truth to tell, most men feel nervous about this too. Though all men and women have sexual fantasies, not everyone feels comfortable about actually trying them. If your partner is not into this and tells you firmly, do not insist. Otherwise, she is liable to walk away from the relationship.

IF A WOMAN SAYS NO…

In any long-term relationship there are bound to be times when your levels of desire are mismatched. Saying no needn't mean rejection, just that one of you is tired, or has had a lousy day. Men are pretty well always ready for sex. But our brains are also somewhat flexible – if a woman signals no, mostly we take the hint (well perhaps one more nuzzle of your neck…) At such times you might understandably feel put down – it just goes to show that men are all ego. Pick up that gripping book again. What is difficult is constant rejection. Then there is a problem.

A thinking man should see that forcing himself on his partner is no basis for a long-term relationship. A man may even start to despise a woman for being subservient. It may be hard, but it is healthier to strive for a relationship where your partner can tell you if she does not want sex and to come to a mutual understanding of the reasons. If you consistently have differing levels of desire, then read page 121 for advice, or talk things over with a professional counsellor.

HOW IMPORTANT IS SEX AND AGE?

Age seems to make little difference to a man's libido, many men still having sex in their seventies, whereas women will often say 'enough' by their sixties.

For most women, sex is an important part of life – but not necessarily the most important part. Most have many other concerns – running a home, pursuing a career, looking after children or elderly parents, and so on. A woman's attitudes to sex are likely to change as she gets older. At nineteen sex can seem the only joy in life; at thirty-five the dual demands of career and children can mean she is constantly knackered, so sex has to take a back seat. After the menopause she might find herself with the time and inclination to start rediscovering her man, but sex will now need to accommodate the physical changes she has undergone. Some women, of course, find sex completely irrelevant, and lead happily celibate lives.

BODY IMAGE

Men and women often feel unhappy about their bodies. A woman may think her tummy is too fat and her breasts are too small. When in bed she may worry that you are fantasizing about some perfect-bodied babe. We all daydream about sex and fantasize a lot, but most of us are able to differentiate between fantasy and reality. There is a great comfort from being with a familiar partner because we know that each of us has realistic expectations about each other. If your partner really were some pneumatic sex goddess, you would probably be in a constant state of worry that some more eligible hunk of a man would carry her off, and if you were a sex god she might have similar worries. Do remember that women can be so touchy about their image that it can be hard for a man to find a tactful way to suggest a bit of weight loss!

I FIND IT HARD TO DISCUSS SEX WITH MY PARTNER

Though embarrassment may be understandable, couples would benefit from being more open about their sex life – especially what gives each pleasure. Men often do not realize that women like sex too and have strong views on what they want. As a last resort your partner might even buy a sex manual and leave it by your bedside. Women's magazines always have articles about sex – she may point one of these out to you. After sex (and before you fall asleep) she might tell you something along the lines of 'that was good, but it could have been even better if…' Be grateful for a really honest statement; do not take it as an assault on your delicate male ego.

THE LOVE DRUG

The biochemistry of lust may not be completely understood, but nevertheless, the proven benefits of sex on our physical health range from the obvious (stress relief), to the more surprising (prostate protection). Just in case you need them, here are a few other reasons to have sex.

- It uses up calories. If you have sex three times a week you'll burn about 7,500 calories per year, which is the equivalent of jogging 75 miles.
- Like all exercise, sex helps lower your cholesterol level.
- Sex boosts your respiratory system. Fast and deep breathing enriches your blood with oxygen, which nourishes your entire body.
- It raises your testosterone levels. Testosterone fortifies bones and muscles. It is a corticosteroid, and its elevation during sex can sometimes reduce the joint inflammation of arthritis.
- Endorphins released during sex are great painkillers – sex can help reduce many minor aches and pains.
- Relaxation at orgasm reduces tension in the neck muscles, thus helping to lessen the frequency of tension headaches.
- Sex delivers a much-hyped hormone called dehydroepiandrosterone (DHEA). In the USA, DHEA's claimed benefits include improving cognition, boosting the immune system, acting as an antidepressant and helping to strengthen bones.
- Sex causes oxytocin to be released; this so-called 'bonding hormone' may have something to do with how inclined we are to show affection, and make us open to hugging, cuddling and touching one another.
- Some prostate problems are aggravated, or even caused, when the fluids in the prostate are not emptied out properly. During orgasm the muscles around the prostate repeatedly contract, forcing out the fluids.
- Sex is a great relaxant, stress reducer and mood improver. Stress and mood both matter medically. If you are relaxed and happy, you are more likely to be healthy than if you are not.

VIAGRA

This intriguing new drug looks set to transform the treatment of impotence; no more need for injections, just take a tablet. Chemically called sildenefil, Viagra has to be taken an hour before intercourse. Soon it will be available as a quick-dissolving wafer that will work more rapidly. Its main side effect is headache. At the time of writing health authorities are still deciding whether Viagra will be obtainable on prescription or only privately.

Sex, lies and misunderstandings

THE IMPORTANCE OF COMMUNICATION

Which of these options would you find easiest?

a) Stripping in front of a woman.
b) Telling her your deepest fears, dreams and ambitions.

a) Painting the kitchen to show your partner you loved her.
b) Telling her you loved her.

If you answered 'a' to either or both of these questions, the chances are you need to take some time to think about your talking and listening skills – that is, about communication.

Communication is not just for wimps. Talking is the only way you can show someone else who you are, what you want, and why you behave as you do. Listening is the only way you can come to understand your partner, and she can learn to understand you. In theory, few people disagree with the claim that good relationships depend on good communication. But it can be difficult to put this belief into practice. Sometimes it is hard to talk, and even harder to listen.

WHAT MAKES GOOD COMMUNICATION?
Good communication requires you to:

- identify your feelings, emotions, fears and ambitions;
- explain these in a way your partner can understand;
- encourage your partner do to the same;
- listen to your partner, and respect her opinions and feelings.

Barriers and benefits

Here are a few examples of common barriers to communication, together with the benefits of overcoming them. The list is not exhaustive, and you will no doubt be able to think up others.

Most barriers to communication are based on fear of one sort or another: fear of intimacy, fear of rejection, fear of looking silly or of growing apart. Overcoming these barriers requires courage – a traditional male virtue.

Barrier: it is scary to reveal our real selves, without keeping anything hidden. It makes us vulnerable to pity, misunderstanding, rejection, and so on.

Benefit: if we have the courage to expose our secret selves to one another, our relationships can only improve since love is partly about trusting another person enough to make ourselves vulnerable, and allowing them to do the same.

Barrier: not saying what you mean – for example, saying that something does not matter, when it does. Or making something else the issue – for example, complaining that you always have to pick up the shopping on the way home from work when what you mean is that you hate your partner working evenings.

Benefit: once your partner knows the general area of the problem (perhaps her career), she can help. She can do nothing about the problem if she believes that nothing is the matter, or senses that something is wrong but has no idea what.

Barrier: we sometimes think it is disreputable for men to have certain feelings, such as feeling insecure or lonely, and for women to have others, such as aggressiveness or daring. This can make it embarrassing to own up to such feelings, or to acknowledge them in a partner.

Benefit: feeling the full range of emotions is part of being a well-rounded, adult human being. Admitting to an emotion not traditionally regarded as masculine will enable your partner to gain a greater insight into your psyche.

Barrier: turning communication into a one-way process – holding forth on some subject without stopping to notice your partner's reaction, changing the subject, being a know-all. All these things can infuriate a woman (and men too).

Benefit: you will circumvent much frustration and anger on your partner's part if you enable her to participate fully in communication.

Barrier: not listening to your partner. This covers a multitude of sins, from half-listening to interrupting, from daydreaming while your partner is speaking, to cutting her off with an abrupt change of subject.

Benefit: by listening to what your partner is saying, you will come to understand her attitudes, beliefs or needs. If you think you have misunderstood, you can always ask for clarification.

Of course, it is much easier to spot barriers to communication when they are written on a page than it is in the fluid give-and-take of everyday life. The task is made harder by the fact that men and women can sometimes badly mislead one another through a variety of mainly unconscious strategies.

The ways we mislead each other

Men and women have different habits and concerns and, especially in the early stages of a relationship, different agendas, perspectives and interests:

- Your partner rings her girlfriends several times a week, even when she has nothing much to say. You never phone your mates like this.
- She tells her friends about her worries and emotions. You talk to yours about sport or work.
- She says, 'you never talk to me', meaning 'you never talk to me about your feelings'. You think, 'what's she on about? I just told her about the great goal I scored in the match today...'
- She wants intimacy, commitment and security; you want sex and freedom.

Such clashes of perspective, acknowledged, unacknowledged or half-acknowledged, lie behind many misunderstandings:

She says: Where's this relationship going?
You think: Help! She wants to know if we should arrange a home birth for our first child.
You say: That girl's pretty.
She thinks: Why's he looking at her? He doesn't love me anymore.

If you want to avoid this sort of misunderstanding, and all the other potential pitfalls to good communication, you and your partner need to work together to:

- identify your individual and joint hopes, desires and needs;
- spell them out to each other in plain and simple terms, taking account of your different perspectives and attitudes.

If you can do this, you should be able to avoid the miseries of suspicion, raised expectations and dashed hopes. Sometimes you'll fail... Most couples row; how they handle their arguments can be a vital indicator of the health of their relationship. We are not talking here about the odd flare-up caused when one of you is feeling bad tempered and wants to pick a fight, but relationship-threatening arguments.

Defusing arguments

All long-term relationships face difficulties, but some situations can lead to particular problems and crises. Examples include:

- difficulties in your sex-life;
- financial problems;
- big contrasts in age or background;
- different attitudes to getting married;
- dissimilar attitudes to having children, or to parenting – especially step-parenting;
- infertility;
- different attitudes to affairs or infidelity.

Of course the problems experienced by a couple in their relationship are unique to their circumstances, and there are no rules for overcoming them. But if your relationship has hit a rocky patch, remember that if you are to survive difficulties as a couple, you must face your problems together. If you find that introducing a difficult topic leads only to shouting, not to a genuine exchange of views and an attempt at resolution, then try to remember some of the following strategies for defusing the situation.

- If things are getting out of hand, call a time-out. Cooling off for ten minutes can give you both time to think about what you really want, and mean.
- Check that you understand what your partner is saying – ask for clarification if necessary.
- Wait to give an opinion, and try to edit what you say. Sometimes silence is a key component in communication.
- Try to inject some humour into the situation – women are usually better at doing this than men, so allow yourself to pick up cues from her.

- Try to avoid 'you' statements – 'you did this, you did that'. Use less threatening 'I' statements instead – 'I really want this, what I meant was that'. 'You' statements tend to blame, 'I' statements describe a situation in neutral terms.
- Try to keep the argument focused – what are you trying to achieve? If you are arguing about money, concentrate on discussing ways you might reduce your monthly outgoings rather than raking over old grudges. Try not to move the goal posts; if you both know what you are trying to achieve, you have a better chance of resolving the situation.
- Shouting, hysteria or crying are sometimes inevitable, but try to remember that we can all control how we express our feelings – even if only to a limited extent.

Defusing strategies may not always work, so remember that disagreements can be useful, since they will help each of you to understand the other's individuality. Respecting your partner's right to have different ideas from you can inject a helpful degree of tolerance into your relationship, and if you explain your own point of view to your partner, she may at least understand you, even if she flatly disagrees with you.

Physical violence

Verbal arguments can sometimes degenerate into physical violence. Perhaps one or other of you simply cannot find the words to express your feelings and violence seems the only way to release tension. Or perhaps one of you was brought up in circumstances where violence was an accepted part of life, so it now seems natural to introduce it into your relationship. Maybe drink or drugs have suppressed the usual internal control mechanisms we all use to monitor our reactions to people and the world around us. If you ever resort to violence as a means to conclude an argument, force your partner to accept your will, vent your feelings, or show your power, then you need to seek professional help as a matter of urgency. You need to do so for yourself, for your partner and for your children if you have any. If you do not get help, not only do you risk losing all sense of self-respect, your loved ones, your home and your career, but you also risk imprisonment. Your GP is a good place to start. He or she will be able to put you in touch with specialist help.

If you are the victim of domestic violence, you may feel you cannot discuss this, because of society's attitudes to women (soft and yielding), to men (hard and aggressive) and to violence (men are the perpetrators, women the victims). But women can be violent and men can be the victims. If this is you, seek help for your partner's sake as well as your own. Once again, your GP is a good place to start.

To summarize

Communication is a big topic, and we have covered it very briefly. But the message should be clear – if you are not used to talking, start now. If you are not used to listening, start now. Your relationship can only benefit, because it is only through talking and listening that we can come to understand one another.

Fertility and contraception

Achieving pregnancy requires fertile sperm, a healthy egg and the nurturing of a fertilized egg in an efficient womb.

SPERM – WHAT YOU NEED TO KNOW

What is a sperm?

It is a single cell packed with genetic material (in the head) and a tail that makes it mobile, plus an energy source below the head. Secretions from the prostate gland activate sperm at the time of ejaculation. When the sperm fuses with an egg it completes the whole genetic code needed to create a new human being.

How many sperm are ejaculated?

Sperm grow within the testicles in enormous numbers. Once fully formed they move away from the testicles into the epididymis (you can feel this behind the testicle) where they live for up to ninety days. The average ejaculate contains between 2–5ml of seminal fluid mixed with sperm. Each millilitre of ejaculate contains millions of sperm – it is normal to have from 50 million to 200 million sperm per ml. At orgasm, all those sperm are thrown inside the vagina, ready to begin their swim towards the egg. So anywhere from 100–1,000 million are deposited, of which just one might be successful.

How do sperm know where to go?

Probably sperm are sensitive to chemical changes within the vagina and womb that lead them on in the right direction to where the egg is in the woman's fallopian tube.

How to separate play from paternity? This simple quest has dogged loving couples as far as we know forever. It is a theological issue too. Is sexual intercourse purely for the purposes of fathering children? Or is it an allowable and pleasurable activity in its own right? While religions vary in their answer to this, modern contraception allows people to make their own decisions – which generally says sex is OK for fun as well as fatherhood.

MALE CONTRACEPTION

Condoms

The simplest contraceptives stop sperm from being deposited in the vagina. The modern condom is a very thin rubber sheath that fits over the penis. The tip is bulbous to act as a reservoir for sperm at the time of ejaculation and the rubber is pre-coated with a lubricant to make it both easy to put on and comfortable during intercourse. As well as being a good contraceptive, condoms also protect against contracting sexually transmitted diseases, as there is no direct genital contact. Tougher condoms are available that suitable for anal intercourse; remember though that this is a high-risk activity for acquiring HIV/AIDS and other sexually transmitted diseases.

How effective are condoms? The best ones are very comfortable and do not interfere with sensation during intercourse. They are 95–98 per cent efficient at preventing pregnancy, a figure which improves if the woman uses a spermicidal cream too. They can be used just when needed and side-effects are unusual (e.g. sensitivity to the rubber or lubricant).

USING A CONDOM

- Always put it on before intercourse as some sperm can leak from the penis even before ejaculation.
- Make sure there is no air in the tip, or the condom may burst.
- Ensure the condom is fully unrolled or sperm may leak out at the base.
- Use a spermicidal cream as well to reduce the risk of conception even more.
- Withdraw soon after orgasm, before the condom slips off the penis as it becomes limp.
- Never re-use condoms; they may be damaged and will have lost lubrication and be contaminated with sperm.

Vasectomy

WHY IS IT DONE?

This is a popular means of contraception, with a high success rate and few serious complications.

WHAT IS INVOLVED?

The sperm leave the testicles via the vas deferens, a tube which you can feel by pressing (gently!) behind your testicles. In a vasectomy both tubes are cut. Under local anaesthetic the surgeon makes a 1cm nick on the scrotum and withdraws the vas, cuts it and ties each end firmly. A stitch closes the cut on the scrotum. Healing takes five to ten days.

AFTERWARDS

It aches for a few days; discomfort, bruising and swelling of the scrotum last from three to seven days but should not get excessive – wearing supportive underpants helps.

HOW SOON DOES IT WORK?

Vasectomy immediately stops sperm getting out of the testicles; but many sperm are stored in the tubes between the testicles and the prostate gland (the vas deferens and epididymis). It takes three to four months for all of these to be expelled during ejaculations. Therefore you must have a sperm count after four months and generally again a month later before being given the all clear. Of course, intercourse can continue during this time but you must keep on using other forms of contraception.

Vasectomy can be reversed by microsurgery with about a 30 per cent chance of success; this is why you should regard vasectomy as a permanent procedure. However, the very latest techniques now allow sperm to be extracted under anaesthetic from the testicle and used for in-vitro fertilization. There is a one in 1,000 chance of the ends of the vas reconnecting spontaneously.

VASECTOMY – SOME COMMON OBJECTIONS
- It hurts like hell – untrue. It aches for a few days.
- It reduces sex drive – no way. Many men find the opposite, knowing that they are safe.
- It causes cancer of the testicles – untrue. This theory has been studied exhaustively, with no scientific evidence found.
- You no longer make sperm – untrue. The testicles carry on production, but the sperm just degenerate and die.

THE FEMALE ORAL CONTRACEPTIVE
WHAT IS IT?
The Pill contains hormones which suppress the woman's own natural menstrual cycle and stop the production of eggs. These hormones are similar to a woman's natural oestrogen (female hormone) and progesterone (hormone for pregnancy). In addition the hormones make the mucus around the cervix (neck of the womb) thicker, making it more difficult for sperm to penetrate. The hormones also make the lining of the womb less receptive to the fertilized egg. The usual pill (the combined pill, containing oestrogen and progesterone) is taken daily for twenty-one days. Then for seven days no pill is taken, during which time the woman has a period. The mini pill (containing progesterone only) has to be taken every day. The rules for taking the pill are complex as is what to do if a woman misses a pill – see manufacturer's literature or speak to your doctor.

OTHER FEMALE CONTRACEPTIVES

The coil
This is the common name for an IUD or IUCD (intrauterine contraceptive device). The coil is a thin plastic device, part of which has copper around it and which is placed inside the womb, where it

can remain for several years. We do not know exactly how it works but it seems to make the lining of the womb reject a fertilized egg.

The diaphragm

This is a dome of rubber – hence its alternative name of the cap – that is inserted by the woman to cover the entrance of the cervix before intercourse. It is about 96 per cent effective at preventing pregnancy. It must be used with a spermicide and left in place for six hours after intercourse to prevent sperm entering the cervix.

Sterilization

The fallopian tubes, along which eggs pass to the womb and by which sperm gain access to eggs, are cut and clipped.

The expectant father

So now she's pregnant. If your relationship is stable, you are both delighted, and the pregnancy seems straightforward – then congratulations! But sometimes life is not quite that simple...

DO YOU BOTH WANT THE BABY?

If the pregnancy was unplanned, it could be that you have very different attitudes to it. It might be that she wants an abortion, but you do not. Or that she wants to keep the baby, but you want her to have an abortion. In this sort of situation, men's rights are non-existent. Despite occasional, high-profile challenges, under British law, the father has no rights over the foetus, and the right to determine the course of the pregnancy lies with the woman. It is irrelevant whether or not the couple is married.

If you do find yourself in either of these situations, then try to get some professional counselling – this is dependent on your partner being willing. Counselling is rarely available on the NHS, although your GP may be able to advise. If you are both under twenty-five, the Brook Advisory Centre can offer help. If you are over twenty-five, the Pregnancy Advisory Service or the Marie Stopes Centre can arrange counselling, although this is not free. Addresses and phone numbers are in the telephone directory.

THE TESTS SHOW SOMETHING'S WRONG

During pregnancy your partner will be offered various screening tests, designed to check on the health and development of your baby. These include tests for Down's syndrome, spina bifida, and normal development of limbs. If they pick up a potential problem, then there will be further diagnostic tests. If these confirm an abnormality, then, depending on its nature and severity, your partner could be offered a termination. Professional counsellors would always be available to help the two of you through this distressing time.

It is worth thinking how, as a couple, you would react to a negative result, before your partner agrees to any tests. They are often presented to a woman as if they are absolutely standard, and she has no choice about whether or not to have them. But there is a choice, and the two of you need to think about whether you want them or not. There is little point in having them if, for example, the two of you share religious objections to abortion.

This is not to deny that having a severely disabled child would place enormous stresses on you, your family and your relationship with your partner. It is merely to point out that it is sensible to consider the issues before, rather than after a negative test result.

TO BE THERE OR NOT TO BE THERE

Do you really want to be there for the birth? If you really would rather not, talk this over with your partner. She may be perfectly happy for you not to attend – there is now such pressure for men to be at the birth that many women feel unable to admit that they don't really want their partner to be present. If she needs persuading, point out to her that 'being there' might not mean being physically present, but rather taking care of the organization of the birth, and later providing her with comfort and a stable environment in which to nourish your baby.

If you have reservations about attending the birth of your child, it is worth considering that other men, who have been in two minds and yet decided to attend, were later very glad that they had been present to support their partner and to welcome their child. Having attended once, few men would miss the birth of any subsequent children.

Is there a way to prepare for this?

For what? For the birth, or for fatherhood? You can prepare for the birth by attending antenatal classes with your partner. But remember, birth, however dramatic and important, is only a finite event; what follows it is in the long term far more important. Before the birth of their first child both women and men can focus so much on labour that they forget this simple fact. Nothing can really prepare you for fatherhood, but you might use the nine months of your partner's pregnancy to read a few child-rearing manuals.

What can I usefully do?

You can, of course, take care of practical details, such as finding a route to the hospital and making sure you've got money for parking. Beyond that, ask your partner what she wants you to do; what one woman regards as useful, another may regard as an insufferable nuisance.

Suppose I make a fool of myself?

What counts as 'making a fool of yourself'? You are unlikely to 'make a fool of yourself' during the early stages of labour, and in the later stages your partner probably will not notice, even if you do. Men do faint sometimes, but your partner will probably forgive you, even if she teases you mercilessly later. Whatever else happens, do resist any temptation to interfere with the actions of the medical attendants. You may want to punch them – don't!

How about if I leave because I can't take it?

Discuss this with your partner before she goes into labour – if you are reluctant to attend the actual birth, this could be a good compromise which she would happily accept.

How should I deal with the new baby?

Do whatever feels most natural to you – a bond will form when you hold your child for the first time, and you gaze into one another's eyes. Try to get involved in the practical aspects of care, such as changing nappies and bath-time. If your partner chooses to breast-feed, remember this is best for your baby and give her your support, even if you are not initially keen. If she opts for mixed breast and bottle or just bottle-feeding, you will be able to help her with this, and should offer to share night feeds. Do not expect life to be a bed of roses – new babies will not let you get any time to yourselves; when once you could go out for an unplanned evening on the town, now even leaving the house will be a major operation. Even if your partner goes back to work, your available income will plummet – a baby is a money pit. In the first few months, sleep deprivation could be a real problem, so you are both likely to be exhausted all the time.

HOW SHOULD I TREAT MY PARTNER, AFTER OUR BABY IS BORN?

Try to admit any troublesome feelings, and do not withdraw into a separate realm, at a time when you and your partner will be in need of each other most. If she is feeling depressed and weepy, deal sympathetically with her state of mind. Try not to be jealous of the bond forming between your partner and the baby, or feel resentful if you think you are no longer Number One in her priorities. The two of you both need time to adapt to the idea that she is no longer simply your partner, but also a mother. Do not force her to fit your preconceived notions of motherhood – do not try to change her 'because that's not how a mother should be'.

You also need time to see yourself as a father and not simply as your partner's partner. This will be easier if you share the day-to-day tasks of caring for a baby – bathing and changing nappies. If your baby is being given a bottle, do some of the night feeds. Helping as much as you can will also serve to lessen any feelings of jealousy you may feel about the way the new arrival seems to consume your partner's affection and time.

WHAT ABOUT OUR SEX LIFE?

If your sex life goes off the boil, don't panic! Survey after survey, as well as anecdotal evidence, show that a couple's sex life is likely to suffer after the birth of a baby. Exhaustion is a factor, as are practical matters, especially if you choose to have your baby sleeping in your bedroom, or even in your bed. For either of you, memories of the birth may also be a deterrent. Your partner could go off sex after childbirth because of pain, or the fear of it. If she is breast-feeding, that could affect your sex life, too.

Babies bring joy, but they also bring a whole new set of headaches. It is barely acceptable to admit this in polite society, which only makes things worse. If you and your partner experience prolonged or serious problems in any area of your relationship after you have become parents, talk to your GP, who will be able to arrange professional counselling, or contact your nearest branch of Relate, who have vast experience in dealing with these problems. Groups such as the NCT (National Childbirth Trust) may also be able to help. (See the phone book for addresses in your area.)

It is quite likely that your partner will feel weepy after the birth; if you suspect her baby blues are tipping into serious depression, talk to your GP. Signs to look for are weeping, neglecting the baby, constant irritability, and expressed (or actual) harm towards herself or the baby.

Male infertility

In 30–40 per cent of cases of infertility it is the man who has the problem. This is why it is essential to have a sperm count before starting infertility treatment for the woman. Do not just assume it is the woman's problem. A normal sperm count should show that you are producing at least 20 million sperm per ml of ejaculate. The sperm should look normal – common abnormalities include a double head, poorly developed tail and poor mobility. If the sperm looks normal, a specialist may perform a post-coital test – that is, sampling sperm from the vagina after intercourse. This shows whether the sperm are surviving, because it can happen that the woman is producing antibodies which are killing off the sperm. Other things to check are:

- Are you having intercourse properly – with penetration and to the point of ejaculation?
- Are you having intercourse regularly, say two to three times a week?
- Is intercourse at the best time of the woman's cycle (around the time of release of the egg which is mid-cycle, about fourteen days from the first day of menstruation in a twenty-eight-day cycle).

For unknown reasons the average male sperm count is falling – the reasons are controversial and not at all established. Infertility is a traumatic event for couples; try to be supportive towards each other and optimistic yet realistic (about 50 per cent of infertile couples will remain infertile).

OTHER FACTORS

You must have your testicles examined. The doctor will check that they are a normal size, and feel at the back for a varicocele (like a collection of varicose veins) which can decrease fertility. Heavy drinking affects fertility (and reduces sexual arousal) as does heavy smoking.

WHAT CAN BE DONE?

You can boost the sperm count by keeping your testicles cooler – wear loose-fitting pants and trousers. Do not have intercourse too often – sperm counts recover over about three days from ejaculation and peak at five to seven days. Alter your technique: try a different position for intercourse that might deliver sperm closer to the cervix (though lying face to face is usually the best for this). Get help for impotence (failure to achieve a satisfactory erection). Some antibiotics may improve sperm counts – doxycycline is one used.

MALE HORMONES

Much mythology surrounds these; they are popular as a boost to libido (sexual desire) and impotence. However, there is no good scientific evidence to support their use, except in the rare cases of true male hormone deficiency, established by sophisticated hormone tests. Whatever benefit men get is probably through a placebo effect.

ARTIFICIAL INSEMINATION

These rapidly changing techniques use your own sperm or donor sperm to fertilize an egg. Fertilization takes place in a test tube (in-vitro fertilization or IVF), and the fertilized egg is then replaced within the woman.

DEALING WITH CHILDLESSNESS

Couples usually feel devastated – men and women; it is one of the hardest issues relationships ever have to face. Both sides feel confused, upset and scared that this problem will force them apart as a couple. Initially they may not want to tell people, or want to be around babies or children. It is natural to need time together to mourn the loss of the children they imagined they would have, and to think about their future as a childless couple. They need to confirm their love for each other, and remember how important it is to hang on to what they have built over their years together.

COMING TO TERMS WITH CHILDLESSNESS

If the whole future is not to be marred by this quirk of biology, then there will come a point when couples just have to accept that nature, even supplemented by technology, is not going to be changed, and allow themselves to move on to the next stage of their lives. Though it may no longer be worth trying for their own child, they can always investigate the possibility of adoption, or fostering. There may be ways in which to channel energies into other forms of creation – artistic or intellectual.

DEALING WITH OTHER PEOPLE'S REACTIONS

You may have to face a variety of crass comments from other people who will tell you to think of all the supposed emotional advantages of remaining childless; how you will have more time for each other, or can develop new interests, and so on. Or they will point out the financial advantages. Or you might have to deal with the fact that other people are speculating about your childless state, especially in the first few years of a partnership. It is worth remembering that most people are genuinely concerned, and want to help. They simply do not know how to, or they may feel embarrassed about raising the subject of children. But there is nothing shameful in infertility, and you should use this fact to give a lead about how you want others to deal with it.

Injecting some spice into your sex life

Here are some suggestions on how you can spice up your sex life, if things seem a little dull.

Perhaps you have been living together for a few years and bed is just somehow going off the boil. A look that once used to say 'Here? Now?' is more likely to be met with 'Dishes? Nappies?' Is this inevitable? What can be done?

The following is to give you some guidance. This cannot be a substitute for a full manual of sexual therapy but it should remove some embarrassment and open some doors. This section is written from a heterosexual viewpoint, i.e. a male/female sexual relationship, and does not explore sex games, sex aids or open sexual relationships. This is not because of prejudice – just a lack of space!

Step 1: review the situation

Sex is important in human relationships but it is only one of many areas of interaction. As relationships develop, sex takes its place among other concerns such as home planning, career development, family, friendship and companionship. Each of these imposes its own pressures, concerns and priorities which may have displaced sex in your thinking.

Where do you each place sex within this wider picture? Do you both agree about its importance or has sex slipped down the agenda for one of you? And however much one of you feels dissatisfied, it is important to know what sex means for your partner. For a man sex can be a simple quick release of tension rather disengaged from emotion. Men can be ready for sex at any time.

For women, on the other hand, sex is more likely to be part of an overall situation of love and care. A day-to-day need for sex is not as common and arousal is more dependent on mood, stress and how well the relationship is going. For a man to ignore this and to insist on sex when he wants is not just insensitive but may even carry legal overtones of marital rape.

Step 2: talk about sex

Your partner cannot guess about how you feel about sex, though in any ongoing relationship she is likely to have a good idea. So talk to her, choosing your moment – as you both rush out the front door in the morning is not the time to say you are feeling sex-starved.

Step 3: confront problems

The commonest sexual problems are premature ejaculation, mismatches of sexual desire (libido), painful intercourse, impotence and failure of orgasm. These may have both physical or psychological causes – for example, impotence may be due to diabetes or depression.

If any of these difficulties is of recent onset, there may be an important physical reason, so see your doctor for a discussion and examination. Assuming physical health is normal, such problems are best dealt with by a sex therapist (though see also Delaying orgasm, below).

Step 4: rediscover each other

This means looking at each other afresh as sexual beings. It is a process of exploring each other's bodies, looking, touching and asking how certain actions feel. Choose a time without interruptions, in a warm place and with the lights on!

One partner looks at the other's body, working their way around the whole body and not just the genitalia. But at the genitalia touch everything to find the most sensitive areas. In a woman, these are likely to be the clitoris, the opening of the vagina especially around the lower half, and the nipples. The position of the clitoris varies greatly between women – remember this as it means that certain positions for intercourse will be more or less arousing than others.

In a man the sexually arousing areas are around the tip of the penis, the underside of the tip and the shaft of the penis, the nipples, and the scrotum.

Step 5: give each other pleasure

The object of this is not necessarily to bring your partner to orgasm, but to see what actions are sexually arousing. You take turns at doing this; it could follow on from the period of inspection given in Step 4 above.

Possibilities are rubbing areas you now know to be sexually arousing, massaging with lotions if this appeals, and licking if you both enjoy this.

All the time you and your partner should be telling each other how it feels, whether to continue or to stop. The object at this stage is not primarily to have penetration or to come to orgasm, but to establish techniques for giving future sexual pleasure. However, it is quite likely that after one or two sessions you will both want to have intercourse as a natural conclusion...

Step 6: delaying orgasm

A common complaint is that the man comes to orgasm before his partner is satisfied. This can be delayed using the well-known squeeze technique. The man has to say or signal that he feels an orgasm is coming. Between thumb and forefinger his partner squeezes the undersurface of the penis just where the tip meets the shaft (technically where the corona meets the frenulum). Keep up the pressure for several seconds, until the penis goes a little limp and the desire for orgasm disappears. This can be repeated as necessary. Women do not require such an active process to stop them coming to orgasm; it should be enough to stop stimulating the clitoris or vagina until the feeling subsides.

Many drugs have been used to delay male orgasm. Alcohol and tranquillizers work for some (but beware not to take so much that you become impotent or simply fall asleep). More sophisticated medication may include low doses of antidepressants (which affect the nerve pathways involved in arousal). SSRIs (selective serotonin reuptake inhibitors, such as Prozac) can reduce sexual desire as a side-effect, which it is possible to put to good use in reducing premature ejaculation.

Step 7: experiment with intercourse

By now you should have a good idea about what you each find arousing and how that leads to orgasm. The actual mechanics of intercourse may seem almost an irrelevance. What you do now depends on your individual preferences. Not every couple wants full intercourse, though most do after bringing the woman to orgasm or to achieve male orgasm.

Step 8: trying different positions

There is a whole literature that suggests that sex can be made more fulfilling by varying the position. There is some truth in this, but less than might be imagined. It is more a matter of comfort and control. Here we describe the advantages and disadvantages of some basic positions. Consult a sex manual for details of variations on each theme.

Man above, woman below:

- Advantages: you face each other, enhancing intimacy and trust. The man is in control of how quickly or slowly he comes. This may be a good position for achieving pregnancy.
- Disadvantages: the woman has no control and might find it difficult to move herself. The depth of penetration can be uncomfortable, depending on the precise position. It is difficult to stimulate the breasts and clitoris.

Woman above, man below:

- Advantages: this is better where the man is heavy; the woman is in control but the man can still stimulate her breasts and clitoris.
- Disadvantages: penetration may be uncomfortably deep for the woman.

Standing or sitting positions:

- Advantages: brings novelty and does not restrict sex to a bedroom setting.
- Disadvantages: requires a degree of gymnastic ingenuity and ability.

Man entering from the rear:

- Advantages: this is a comfortable position to use in later pregnancy. It allows the man to caress the clitoris or breasts during intercourse.
- Disadvantages: it is not as intimate in terms of looking and speaking to each other.

There are no right or wrong positions as long as sex remains comfortable for both partners and each achieves satisfactory pleasure and orgasm. Changing positions is a quick way to enhance your lovemaking but is not a substitute for the mutual trust and pleasuring of foreplay mentioned earlier.

MYTHOLOGY ABOUT SEX

I'm not having as much sex as everyone else

The facts about who is having it, and how often, are difficult to establish. As a very rough guide well under 10 per cent of couples have sex every day, about another 50 per cent have sex at least once a week, about 20 per cent have sex once or twice a month. The rest either no longer have sex or have it more infrequently or are not prepared to tell an interviewer!

A woman who does not reach orgasm during intercourse is unfulfilled

This a hoary debate, based on a theory of two types of female orgasm, that from stimulation of the clitoris and that from stimulation of the vagina during intercourse. Reliable data is even more difficult to obtain, with women who always have orgasms varying from about 15–50 per cent, those who never have orgasms from about 4–30 per cent, and others having orgasms sometimes or often. It is better to concentrate on the overall quality of lovemaking rather than to aim to achieve orgasm during intercourse.

Mutual masturbation is not 'real' sex

Though not full penetrative sex, this can be a deeply pleasurable experience nevertheless. Sex therapists agree that being able to bring each other to orgasm successfully is an important part of dealing with sexual problems in relationships, because it shows how partners can find out what gives satisfaction and how to control it.

We can't have sex at our age

Undoubtedly sexual activity declines with age but this does not mean it disappears. Some women report increased libido after the menopause. Many men and women have continuing sexual desires well into old age. The mechanics may need adjusting to take account of stiff joints, painful hips and reduced female lubrication but there are ways round all these. For many couples sex, however occasional, remains a comforting reaffirmation of their love.

Programme for change

Part Two of this book has been about getting the most from your relationship, about how you can increase your levels of communication and of sexual satisfaction to the benefit both of yourself and of your partner. If both of you sense you need and want to make changes in your relationship, you could start by working through this programme for change together.

Sometimes, you may need the help of a trained therapist to identify relationship problems or, having identified them, to help you tackle them. If you feel you would benefit from such help, contact your nearest branch of Relate (listed in the phone directory).

Step 1: identify what you want to change

Are you most concerned about changing destructive patterns of jealous behaviour, about practical problems, about the lack of variety in your sex life, about the fact that you have differing levels of desire for sex...or what?

Only the two of you together can decide what you want to change. Start by sitting down and talking through potentially problematic areas. Make sure that as well as talking, each of you listens to the other.

Let's take Sally and Mike as an example. Sally is in her early thirties, Mike is ten years older. They have been living together for just over a year and are unmarried. Both have demanding careers, and neither wants children at the moment, although Mike has an eight-year-old son from a previous marriage.

Sally thinks that since she moved in with Mike he has started taking her for granted sexually: 'He never makes any effort to please me any more. He treats me like his sister, rather than his partner.'

After a great deal of prompting Mike was prepared to admit that he did find sex with Sally somewhat unexciting these days, although he still loved her, and wanted to be with her.

Step 2: set your priorities

In this area of your life, deciding on the problem and setting priorities are likely to merge into one. In a nutshell, the problem for Sally and Mike was that familiarity breeds boredom, and their priority was to prevent boredom from moving up a notch into contempt.

Step 3: identify potential obstacles

By identifying their problem, Sally and Mike had already overcome the main obstacle to beating it. It took courage on both their parts to own up to this difficulty in their relationship. Mike especially felt disloyal in owning up to finding sex somewhat unexciting, and Sally needed great strength of character to try to see this admission in a positive light.

How could they overcome this depressing sense of familiarity? They decided on two main steps:

- To go out and do interesting things together, go to the theatre, see friends, attend sports events, etc., to give them outside stimulation and new topics of conversation.
- To explore some of Mike's fantasies: 'I'd always wanted to see Sally in rubber gear, but never dared ask her. But when I did put it to her, she was enthusiastic, so we decided to give it a go.'

Step 4: set a timetable

You may not think that it is appropriate to set a formal timetable for results when tackling relationship problems. But some sense of time pressure might be helpful. Sally and Mike felt that if they were still dissatisfied after six months of really working on their relationship, then they might be unable to resolve their problems alone, and would seek professional help.

Step 5: review progress

In order to review progress, we suggest you keep a diary specifically for this purpose. Jot down anything which seems relevant to your chosen aim. For example, a few weeks after they had initially talked, an entry in Sally's diary read: 'We seem to be well on the way to overcoming the staleness we felt. The stimulation of going out together so much really helps – I think it's good for Mike to see me talking, joking, even flirting with other people. It makes him see me in a sexy light.'

If you feel you are making no headway, re-motivate yourself by reminding yourself why you embarked on the programme for change, and the positive benefits you are aiming to achieve...your relationship is worth improving, or saving. Remember, you might need to get the professional advice of a trained therapist.

Step 6: reward achievement

When it comes to trying to improve your relationship, why not reward effort, rather than waiting to reward achievement? To reward Mike for joining her in confronting their problems, Sally decided to give him his birthday present a few weeks early, and presented him with a season ticket for his local football club. Meanwhile Mike resolved not to let Sally feel taken for granted again. He started by devoting an evening to staying in with her so they could talk about aspirations – hers and theirs.

If you fail in your attempts to improve your relationship, but you both feel there is something to save, do not despair. You did well to try, and you can always try again...with good will on both parts you should succeed next time.

PART THREE
mental
HEALTH

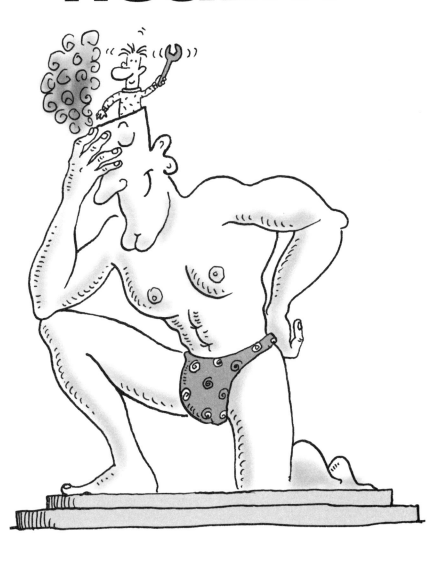

The basics

YOUR MENTAL HEALTH: WHY WORRY?

Browse through your daily paper. Chances are that there will be at least one report about someone quitting their job through stress. They may even be suing their employer for subjecting them to unreasonable pressure. For every case which hits the papers, there are thousands more circumstances which people just put up with, or which at worst, lead to problems such as:

- quiet misery;
- deteriorating job performance;
- personal unhappiness;
- family stresses or breakdown;
- turning to alcohol, drugs or tranquillizers.

Men who encounter more serious mental health problems might find themselves experiencing depression, agoraphobia (a fear of meeting new people and severe anxiety in social settings), or the complete inability to cope, popularly called a nervous breakdown (more properly called an acute stress reaction).

These emotions are common; severe anxiety is estimated to affect up to one person in twenty while milder but significantly uncomfortable anxiety affects up to 15 per cent of the adult population. Other serious mental illnesses are also remarkably common. Schizophrenia affects about one person in every 200, severe depression about one person in every fifty to 100. More people than you might imagine suffer from phobias such as agoraphobia.

Imagine what this means. Look around your office or place of work. Of every six people you see, probably one has a significant anxiety problem. You might wonder whether this matters to you – but it certainly should. The person who snaps back at you or leaves work unfinished or who upsets customers may be doing this through the effects of stress. And that can rebound on you, in terms of adding to your workload, forcing you to sort out problems, quite apart from the sheer unpleasantness from working in a stressed environment.

You are part of everyone else's environment; so if you are also having mental health difficulties, they will rebound on your colleagues just as their difficulties affect you. And do not forget your potential. You could become a hero; do not be one with a fatal flaw.

One more thought: do you really want to live in an uncaring setting, where everyone else's problems are their problems alone?

MENTAL HEALTH: THE THREATS TO YOU

The cosy men's club in employment is breaking down. Good thing too. But do not forget men are not women; their psychology is different. Men:

- prefer to do rather than think;
- prefer to keep emotions under control rather than expressing them;
- tend to regard anxiety or inability to cope as being a reflection of personal weakness, rather than being a natural emotion and experience;
- would rather talk about sport than stress.

The world is still dominated by men and male psychology still prevails. This means that men are expected to:

- get on with things, regardless of other pressures;
- not make a fuss;
- ignore physical or mental symptoms for longer than women might;
- resist other people's emotional demands or weaknesses;
- not say how they feel, not confide and definitely not cry.

This all forms what we recognize as the macho male persona. Action man, all doing and little thinking or emotion. Like all stereotypes, action man is an exaggeration. Plenty of men are sensitive to others' emotional status, while being a women is no guarantee of being receptive to others' feelings. But as a broad generalization, the above is a fair interpretation of male psychology.

Workaholism and burn-out

Given the typical male mental settings, it is not too surprising that they are liable to these problems. As we might say: 'Do you want to reach your potential? Do you want to keep firing on all cylinders and perform at peak efficiency? Do you want to work until you decide to quit and not until life waves you goodbye?'

Workaholism may affect someone you already know. A colleague perhaps, or could it be you? The workaholic is not odd or obsessive; rather they are typically conscientious and good at their job. They get a buzz from doing things right, getting the contract, doing the business, designing the project. They are probably enthusiasts in other spheres of their life. As they so often like to put it, 'If the job's worth doing, it's worth doing well.' Who can argue with that? And some presumably are workaholics through a desire to avoid other aspects of their life, such as their partners and families.

So it happens that a job demands working later than usual or getting in earlier than normal. It may require some evening work or even weekend work. But, they say to themselves, this is a one-off for this special project. Still there is no denying the kick they get from the successful completion and the rewards that may accompany it by way of approval, bonus, promotion or pay.

Soon another 'special project' presents itself and they spend more time on it. The success, the acclaim, and the rewards of satisfaction feed on themselves. Before long they are working all hours; work takes priority over the rest of their family or personal life.

Though the workaholic may feel under pressure, the pressures are to a large extent self-imposed. They do not necessarily feel stressed. This is how being a workaholic differs from simply being overworked and under stress. The person under stress from work seeks to avoid it, whereas the workaholic seeks for more.

ARE YOU A WORKAHOLIC?

- Do you always put work first?
- Do you feel that a work crisis must take priority over a domestic crisis?

- Do you regularly take work home in the evenings and at weekends?
- Do you work over and beyond what the job really demands?
- Do you seek out extra work?
- Do you not take all your holidays?
- Do you ring into work even when you are on holiday?
- Do you wonder why you are reading this rather than working?

Workaholism: is it all bad?

Of course not. The world relies on people who give over and beyond the average, people who are building new enterprises and striving for perfection. Success and progress more than ever rely on hard work, long hours and constant purposeful activity. A hero in fact...

So is it all good?

It can be, as long as the workaholic's priorities are reasonably in line with the priorities of the 'significant others' in their life. Within the work setting this will probably taken for granted; work is built and thrives on enthusiasm and energy. But this may not necessarily be the case within family and social life. Your domestic partner may share your workaholic outlook because she wants to share in the rewards it brings. But your children may not. And there comes a point in even the most successful lifestyle where others say 'enough'. Or perhaps the rewards fail to materialize after a point. You become known as 'the guy who will get things done', so things get passed to you and others expect you to do them, but without reward. If so, it is time for a major review of your life.

If you think all the time about work, or if your sleep is disturbed by thinking about work, workaholism may be getting out of hand. If this is what you are experiencing, you should re-evaluate your lifestyle. Consider the strategies given below in Burnout.

BURNOUT

This appears to be a recent phenomenon though perhaps it is just a new word for an old problem. We recognize people who have reached a certain position in their career, who have been effective and are full of ideas but whose performance starts to go off the boil. It eventually becomes clear that this is not through lack of motivation or ability but rather through a change in their mental outlook.

Burnout can affect people at any age, though it is classically associated with people in their early forties. People at this age should be at the peak of their careers in terms of ability, health, energy, knowledge, professional standing, economic and personal stability. When their performance declines, it stands out starkly and it is reasonable to ask why.

People make all sorts of excuses for burnout. It does not mean physically being no longer able to cope with stress, nor losing the edge, nor loss of youthful eagerness and openness to change, nor getting fed up with a job through boredom. Although these are common symptoms (see below), they are not the cause but the effect.

Burnout – some symptoms

- The enthusiasm for all aspects of the job diminishes.
- There is resistance to any change and any new ideas.
- There is a feeling of pointlessness about the job.
- There is a reluctance to plan ahead, especially where it involves more change.
- Sufferers become irritable with clients and colleagues.
- Time gets spent on unimportant tasks at the cost of ignoring more urgent priorities.
- There is an increase in tiredness and time taken for illness.

Theories of burnout

- It is just getting realistic about where you are in life and where you are likely to go.
- It is because the economic pressure to perform is reduced.
- It is only a natural fact of ageing to which psychologists have given a fancy name.
- It affects old buffers who can't cope and should get out.
- It happens because you realize that there is more to life than work.

WORKAHOLISM AND BURNOUT – WHAT CAN YOU DO ABOUT THEM?

- Think about what your job means to you. Write down what aspects you enjoy, which you can put up with and which you find unacceptable.

- Consider whether your job can be adjusted to make it more in line with your preferences.
- Discuss with colleagues how you feel – they may well be feeling the same (that male macho thing again...)
- Can you reduce your working hours, shed some responsibility, or opt out of certain aspects of your work?
- Can you take time out to get things in perspective – take a holiday or a sabbatical?
- Try to develop hobbies and outside activities that could give you the satisfaction you no longer get from work.

If these fail, the choices become starker – leave the job, change the job or alter your life altogether. Is this opting out? Not at all; some people would say that this is the truly heroic way to cope with burnout.

Coping with change and insecurity

Like it or not, change is a fact of life for the foreseeable future. Few people relish this; routines are comfortable, become automatic and get honed to a reasonable degree of efficiency. But outside pressures are bound to interfere, perhaps in the form of automation, take-overs, legislation or competition. You may be one of the heroes affecting the changes! Or you may be one of those facing redundancy and job loss. Here are some suggestions to help you to cope.

- Accept the inevitable; do not turn a blind eye to coming changes, they will not go away and when changes do come others will be seen to be better prepared, co-operative and enthusiastic.
- Participate in planning. Many dumb things get done in the name of change. Make this less likely by getting involved in the planning; this can be an opportunity for you to enhance your standing, because you will be able to demonstrate an expertise and knowledge of your job your superiors may never have been aware of.

- Ask for training. Again, this will enable you to overcome the fear of the unknown and makes it less likely that any problems on Day One of the changes will reflect badly on you.
- Ask for feedback. You cannot be expected to cope with major changes immediately and smoothly. Get feedback on how you are doing; turn this into a quality exercise by relaying back those aspects of the changes which in your view need adjusting.
- Talk about how you feel, sharing your natural feelings of insecurity, uncertainty and frustration. Go on, you are a hero, you can do it. But make a distinction between discussing changes in a supportive and constructive way as opposed to simply condemning them (unless you really are prepared to put your head on the line).
- Keep a sense of humour.
- Sympathize with your bosses; chances are they no more like the need for change than you do.

CAN A HERO BE ASSERTIVE WITHOUT BEING AGGRESSIVE?

This is possible and is an important strategy to learn if you feel that work is tending to dominate other aspects of your life. The skills are useful in other settings too, where you want to put your view across firmly. The steps involved are:

- Feeling positive about yourself and feeling confident in your right to act or think as you do.
- Make sure your body language is positive – sit or stand upright; keep eye contact; speak firmly and clearly but not necessarily loudly; use phrases which are positive, such as 'I feel that' or 'I would like to' or 'We could consider doing...'
- Learn to avoid weak phrases such as 'Could you perhaps...' or 'Maybe you could...'
- Repeat your requests or thoughts calmly until you feel the other party has heard and understood what you are saying.
- Avoid shouting and gesturing, and insulting or demeaning language.
- Learn when and how to compromise without forcing either side to lose face.

Mental health – additional problems

The above is an introduction to mental health. You will find many specialized texts and organizations to help you further. Now we will consider some other common mental health problems that all men (and women) are bound to face.

STRESS

Stress is a concept borrowed from mechanics: if too much stress (that is pressure or force) is placed on part of a machine, then the part is weakened and may even break, and the machine no longer functions at maximum efficiency. It is not so different from a psychological point of view – if you are subject to continual stress (unmanageable forces in your life) then your ability to cope is undermined, and you can no longer perform at your best.

The mind affects the body, and stress boosts production of the two hormones adrenaline and noradrenaline. In the short term these chemicals, together with others called corticosteroids, are responsible for an increase in breathing and heart rates, tensed muscles and queasiness. This is the so-called 'fight or flight response', which was useful in stressful situations in the dim evolutionary past – when we needed to flee predators. But nowadays, the fight or flight response is frequently produced in inappropriate, evolutionary unimportant circumstances, such as a traffic jam, or a business meeting. Prolonged exposure to the chemicals produced under stress can lead to a range of physical symptoms – anything from allergies to impotence, or insomnia to muscle pains.

This is not to say that stress is necessarily a bad thing. Stress is a natural part of life and we all need a little of it to provide us with the motivation to challenge our limits, overcome obstacles or aim for the top. Positive stress offers us healthy stimulation, and life would be dull without it. Problems arise only when stress levels exceed an individual's ability to cope, and begin to have a negative impact on life. The trick with stress is to learn how to manage it, not to try to banish it altogether.

Your stress personality

Tolerance of stress varies from individual to individual. Some men get a rush from taking risks; they thrive on stress. They are the ones who work eighty-hour weeks and have a stream of women on tap. Others succumb much more easily to pressure and stress-related disorders. They are the ones who lie awake at night worrying about the mortgage and who prefer a stable working environment.

This suggests that we might all reveal different stress personalities, and indeed it is sometimes claimed that there are four principal types of stress personality: mellow, compensatory, frustrated and hyper. Use the following table to identify your own stress personality. Perhaps you fall between two categories; if so, keep a note of both. Later in this section you will need to know your stress personality in order to choose natural remedies to help you cope with stress.

	Mellow	Compensatory	Frustrated	Hyper
Energy level when stressed	No energy	Erratic energy	Low energy	Excessive energy
Thinking power when stressed	Difficulty in concentration	Distraction and short-term memory loss	Scattered and erratic thoughts	Scattered thoughts and loss of listening skills
Physical symptoms when stressed	Fatigue, lethargy and excessive sleeping. Overeating	Muscle tension and headaches	Constipation and other digestive disorders	Insomnia and restlessness
Mental reactions when stressed	Depression and persistent negative thinking	General dissatisfaction, and hypersensitivity to criticism	Anxiety and persistent worrying – especially about others	Anxiety, anger and aggressiveness. Compulsive behaviour
When stressed I tend to…	Drink alcohol (a depressant)	Get involved in excessive social activity	Drink caffeine (a stimulant)	Use sex to relieve tension

Stress triggers

Some situations are recognized to be stress triggers, whatever the victim's stress personality. Many of these triggers are to do with losing control – if you feel in control of your life, you are less likely to be stressed, whereas if you feel that you cannot control events, or that others are controlling you, you are more likely to be stressed.

Stress triggers can be organized in different ways; psychologists sometimes use a system based on so-called internal and external triggers. Here we use a slightly different approach. Most triggers fall into four broad categories:

- money and work;
- temperament and health;
- relationships;
- lifestyle.

IDENTIFYING YOUR OWN STRESS TRIGGERS, AND TAKING ACTION

If you have lost control in some area of your life, and are thus feeling stressed, the first step towards remedying the situation is to identify your stress triggers. Perhaps you have already done this – you know that your unreasonable boss is placing impossible demands on you, and that this is making you stressed. But perhaps you merely feel stressed, and don't know why. If so, the grid below should help you identify the problem.

Think about how many of these triggers apply to you. Wherever feasible, for each trigger we have also included an action plan for regaining control. Of course, the triggers we have identified may not exactly map your circumstances. If this is the case, use our grid as a template for drawing up your own. For each trigger you identify in your own personal grid, it is important also to draw up an action plan, with the aim of regaining control of your life.

Dealing with stress

A range of relaxation techniques can be employed to help overcome the negative effects of stress – see page 148 or the Appendix. Choose a technique which suits you, and try to incorporate it into your regular routine. On page 210 we talk about the importance of breathing consciously in a way intended to reduce stress. Even if you try nothing else, it is worth mastering this technique, as it can be employed at any time, and in any place, whenever stress threatens to overwhelm you.

Regular exercise, a healthy diet and decent sleep all contribute to stress management. See page 25 for advice on exercise, page 13 for advice on diet and page 35 for tips on overcoming insomnia.

Natural remedies

Natural remedies can be excellent stress-busters. In the following table, we have tailored suggestions to the stress personalities outlined above. If you fall between two personalities, experiment with suggestions for each. For more detailed advice specific to your needs, consult a qualified therapist.

	Herbs	Homoeopathy	Manipulative therapy	Other
Mellow	Ginseng boosts energy. St John's wort helps alleviate depression	Take natrum carbonicum for exhaustion and melancholy	Swedish massage can counteract depression	Yoga or T'ai chi can overcome lethargy and exhaustion
Compensatory	Try hops or valerian for insomnia; skullcap or feverfew for headaches	Pulsatilla may help insomnia, headaches and general touchiness	Chiropractic can help with tension and headaches	Aromatherapy – ylang-ylang can help balance erratic energy (do not take internally)
Frustrated	Camomile and peppermint are good for the digestive system	Argentum nitricum can help relieve excessive worry about loved ones	Shiatsu can help relieve anxiety	Flower remedies – white chestnut is good for obsessive worrying
Hyper	Hops or valerian are calming	Nux vomica is useful if you get over-critical, angry and competitive under stress	Cranial osteopathy can help calm aggressive moods	Acupuncture could help you balance mood swings and anger

Stress triggers

MONEY AND WORK

● **BEING IN DEBT**
Action: talk to your bank about re-financing your debt. If you owe money to more than one lender, it might be possible to take out a single loan to pay them all off – this would be cheaper than having many loans.

● **BEING BADLY PAID**
Action: negotiating yourself a pay-rise will take time and effort. Start by scanning the job adverts relevant to your work, so you are sure of the going rate. If you are genuinely underpaid, point this out to your boss, but do not expect immediate action.

● **HAVING AN UNREASONABLE BOSS**
Action: if your boss is a pig, and is making totally impossible demands, could you take your complaint over his head? Or transfer out of his department? Or would he be amenable to the idea of hiring an extra member of the team to take the pressure off you?

● **UNCERTAINTY OF EMPLOYMENT**
Action: that there are no longer jobs for life has its upsides. Remind yourself that you are not shackled to one firm for life; you can take your skills and sell them to the highest bidder. If unemployment strikes, it is not a social disaster, nor a cause for shame – it is just another phase in your career.

TEMPERAMENT AND HEALTH

● **BEING A NATURAL WORRIER**
Action: try to remind yourself how much time is wasted by worrying, and how many worries come to nothing. This is unlikely to stop you worrying in the short term, but might help you get your worries in proportion in the long term.

● **BEING QUICK-TEMPERED OR IMPATIENT**
Action: if you feel you are about to lose it, take a few deep breaths and count to ten – old advice, but useful. Tell yourself that losing your temper will send your blood pressure shooting up, which can only be bad for you.

● **BEING DEPRESSIVE**
Action: why not talk to your GP? He or she will not think less of you for facing up to your depression, and could offer much needed support and help.

● **SUFFERING A LONG-TERM HEALTH PROBLEM**
Action: whatever the specific details of your problem, try to draw up an action plan for coping, or managing, especially during a crisis. Join a self-help group, and read everything you can about your problem – knowledge is power.

Stress triggers

RELATIONSHIP

● **GETTING MARRIED**
Action: planning a wedding can be deeply stressful. Remind yourself that the stress will only be short-lived, and that it is probably better to accept compromises now than sow the seeds for long-term family grievances.

● **SPLITTING UP**
Action: do not try to hide the way you are feeling from friends and family, and if you feel you are not coping, get some professional help – from Relate, for example.

● **BECOMING A PARENT**
Action: in the first few months after your baby is born, make sure you keep lines of communication open with your partner.

● **BEREAVEMENT**
Action: the death of a spouse, a child, a close relative or a friend will be harrowing. Do not be too proud to accept offers of help. Try to stay in regular touch with friends and family. If you feel you cannot cope, get some professional help, perhaps from Cruse (an organization to help the bereaved, see Useful Addresses).

LIFESTYLE

● **COMMUTING AND LONG HOURS**
Action: commuting, especially on over-crowded roads and trains, is stressful. Assuming you have investigated all alternative methods of getting to work, could you perhaps work from home one or two days a week? This might also solve the problem of long hours, since you could probably accomplish twice as much while at home, than when surrounded by all the distractions of the office.

● **MOVING HOUSE**
Action: in the olden days, people did not move, or at least not very far and not very often. Now people move all the time, and the whole experience is stressful, right from putting your property on the market, to unpacking your bags in the new place. However hard, try to maintain a positive attitude, and think how happy you will be when finally you are settled. Remind yourself this is short-term stress.

● **NOISE AND CROWDING**
Action: those of us who live in cities are constantly bombarded by noise, and by other people. If this is you, try to get out of the city once in a while, to re-charge your batteries.

ANXIETY

You feel anxious; what does this mean? Anxiety means worry which is mingled with fear. The fear may be of a very specific nature – perhaps tomorrow you have a job interview, or a review of your performance at work or a meeting with a new client. Your mind roves over the possible ways in which things could go wrong, to the exclusion of things that could go right.

Or perhaps there is not so much a definite source of worry but you just feel anxious in general. This so-called free-floating anxiety is a vague sense of fear that will attach itself to any convenient hook. The car makes an odd sound and you think 'Oh no, what could that be?' Then your partner makes a remark that you take to be a criticism and you cannot get worry about that out of your head.

Strictly speaking, worry means anxiety attached to a couple of specific problems, whereas anxiety is a more diffused free-floating emotion. But in practice the states overlap, together with elements of stress and even depression.

What does anxiety do?

Anxiety uses up energy, as do all strong emotions. Instead of this energy going into constructive thought and planning, your mind keeps returning to the same topics, squeezing out the goal-directed thoughts that should be following more useful channels.

Psychological effects

Anxious people feel tired, often complain of headaches and can expect disturbed nights. They find that they cannot concentrate on a task at hand for long – soon anxiety breaks their concentration. They may feel their memory is affected, when really it is that same lack of concentration which is to blame. They may lose interest in sex (loss of libido). Being on edge, they become irritable and have a short fuse. In the most severe anxiety states you lose the ability to function at all. Work and home life get neglected because either you feel too anxious to start anything or whatever you do start you are easily distracted from some other more worrying job.

Physical effects

The list is enormously long. The commonest symptoms are sweating, a mild tremor of the hands, aching across the shoulders from tense muscles, fidgeting and twitches. That aching often extends up the neck into the head and is thought to explain why anxiety causes headaches. You may get palpitations (awareness of the heartbeat), feel breathless (typically unable to breathe deeply enough), have a dry mouth and feel difficulty in swallowing. Indigestion, diarrhoea and stomach cramps are common.

ANXIETY: A CHECK LIST
How many of the following symptoms are you experiencing?

- Feeling you need more air to breathe.
- Over-breathing.
- Tremor of your hands.
- Headaches.
- Aching muscles, especially your shoulders and neck.
- Dry mouth.
- Loose motions/diarrhoea.
- Feeling a lump in your throat on swallowing.
- Palpitations.
- Aching in your chest.
- Needing to pass urine frequently.
- Failure of erection.

Do you experience four or more of these? If so, it is most likely that you are in an anxiety state. But see below for other medical possibilities.

Not all anxiety is from anxiety

Anxiety is so common that it is tempting to ascribe many vague symptoms to it. There are a couple of conditions in particular that can mimic anxiety in a younger person; these are an overactive thyroid gland and depression. These should be suspected if you are also experiencing weight loss, increased appetite or anxiety mingled with gloom and loss of joie de vie (see also Depression, page 150). Heart, lung and digestive problems may produce similar symptoms, too. However the more symptoms you have, the more likely anxiety is to blame. See your doctor for an opinion.

Anxiety triggers

The fear aspect of anxiety often attaches to specific areas. For example, agoraphobia is an anxiety about going out into public places, and claustrophobia is a fear of being in a confined space (such as a lift). These are phobias – fears attached to a specific object or situation. Some people get panic attacks; additional stress sets off overwhelming anxiety, sweating and all-embracing fear. You may feel unable to leave the house or you suddenly have to stop driving.

Is anxiety a good or a bad thing?

In fact it is both. Without some degree of anxiety, hundreds of things would be left undone. A degree of stress in our lives is a motivator. But you probably would not be reading this section unless you felt that the anxiety in your life was getting out of hand. And if you would rather not take notice because you think it is weak, you should realize that severe anxiety will be eventually be noticed by others and may affect your career.

Anxiety – weakness or misfortune?

SOME ARE BORN THAT WAY…

Some people are naturally anxious personalities; throughout life they are subject to worry and fears. This type of anxiety often runs in families.

SOME ACHIEVE IT…

These are the workaholics of this world who seek ever more demanding challenges and who push themselves to a point where all the balls are up in the air – and poised to fall on their heads (see Workaholism and burnout on page 133).

AND SOME HAVE IT THRUST UPON THEM…

Others develop anxiety through abnormal stresses. This can happen to any of us under the right (actually wrong) pressure and does not reflect on you as being a weak individual. In fact it is often the conscientious individual trying to do his best who is most affected, by stresses which are just too demanding for him. Such work or socially imposed stress is a major component of the increased anxiety in our society, especially for people who are faced with constant change and a feeling of not being in control of their circumstances.

ARE PARENTS TO BLAME?
Psychological theories of anxiety do put the blame on childhood upbringing. The truth of this is highly debatable. If your childhood was unstable, it seems logical that it would lead you to be an anxious adult. Yet it is possible to argue the other way round; that uncertainty in childhood leads the adult to seek security. Psychotherapy does often help people with anxiety, so there may be more to such theories than at first impression.

Strategies for coping with anxiety

This is going to sound like a mixture of common sense and the obvious. Do not dismiss it for these reasons.

1 List the various symptoms you might have been feeling (see Anxiety checklist on page 145). Add this list of symptoms to the additional possibilities above.
2 Accept that your anxiety is a real problem.
3 Review the stresses in your life. For at least four weeks, keep a note of situations which cause anxiety, putting down what you identify as the cause. Analyse your notes for patterns. Does anxiety occur on particular days of the week, times of day or during specific tasks, situations or when you are with certain individuals?
4 Allocate priorities to these anxiety-rich situations, i.e. are there some which are completely unavoidable, such as an examination, as compared to others less urgent, such as a date to start golf lessons. Only you can decide how to arrange the priorities.
5 Now write about anything which you have found relieves anxiety. Possibilities might include sports, meeting friends, having a drink, cigarettes, drugs, sex or entertainment. Analyse each of these. Are they realistic options or are they self-destructive? Narrow down the choice to things which will enhance your life as well as relaxing you.
6 Can you rearrange your job to reduce stress? Could you could renegotiate your work, reallocate priorities, delegate more, become more assertive about deadlines, working hours, or pressures imposed on you? (See also Burnout on page 133). There may even be simple changes you could introduce such as a better chair or a quieter office.

7   Is your life going where you want it to? Are there priorities which
have got lost in the day-to-day mayhem. Consider how realistic it
is for you to redirect yourself towards your goals.

Relaxation techniques

Any or all of the following might be right for you. The advantage is
that you can do them on your own. No one else need be aware of
your supposedly guilty secret. In fact, your job competitor may
already be practising these...

Learn brief relaxation techniques to use several times a day. For
example, take perhaps just two minutes in which to breathe slowly
and deeply while consciously thinking about tension in your various
muscle groups and willing them to relax. Other variations involve
visualizing a favourite and soothing experience or scene, thinking
yourself through all aspects – the sights, smells and tastes.

MEDITATION

This also requires you to start by relaxing all your muscles. Then
breathe slowly and deeply, while repeating a selected phrase or
word to yourself, continuing for up to twenty minutes.

EXERCISE

This is an excellent relief for anxiety, and it works in several ways. By
removing yourself from the anxiety-provoking environment, you
divert attention away from your worries. Exercise also generates a
hormonal effect through the release of endorphins – natural brain
chemicals with relaxing properties. Physical activity could range
from gardening through walking to swimming and jogging. Steady
exertion seems to be more beneficial than brief energetic activities
such as a workout at a gym.

HELP FROM OUTSIDERS

You will probably need to get support from others if anxiety
dominates your life to the extent that your family, friends and
colleagues begin to comment on its effects. If you've tried the self-

help above, and tried to analyse your situation in order to improve it, but things remain unclear, overwhelming or too painful to confront – then you should consider outside help. There are various options.

TALKING ABOUT SYMPTOMS

Remarkably, simply having it explained that anxiety can be the cause of symptoms may be enough. It further helps if the explanation comes from a trusted adviser, be that your doctor, counsellor or perhaps a friend or partner. This is especially the case where you have troubling physical symptoms from anxiety – things such as tension in your neck, over-breathing or palpitations. It often also helps in such cases to have a physical check-up to put your mind at rest about the state of health of your heart, lungs and blood pressure. After explanation, you might be able to turn again to the relaxation techniques mentioned earlier.

RELAXATION WORK

This more formal help teaches you techniques of relaxation such as deep breathing and muscle relaxation. You might feel somewhat stupid practising deep breathing on your own; go to a class to see how helpful it can be and that you are not alone in your mental tension.

PSYCHOTHERAPY

This is the heavy stuff – it is relatively rarely necessary, though very useful if needed. Consider it where anxiety is resistant to the other self-help measures and especially where you yourself suspect that the roots of the anxiety lie with deep-seated experiences and worries.

Be prepared for a long and bumpy ride. You will need at least six hours of discussion even for brief psychotherapy. That can be enough to explore childhood influences, or longstanding relationship problems.

The type of psychotherapy is a matter of personal preference. Psychoanalytic therapy (emphasizing any deep-seated unhappiness or insecurity about yourself and possible childhood sexual conflicts) is falling from favour. The current 'in' therapy is cognitive therapy, whereby you try to rethink the way you see the world and thereby to think yourself out of the roots of anxiety. In a nutshell, this is the power of positive thinking.

TRANQUILLIZERS AND SEDATIVES

You will find that doctors hesitate to prescribe these drugs. Where they do agree to do so, it will be for short courses (a couple of weeks) to see you over the worst of your anxiety. Drugs used include benzodiazepines such as diazepam. Their advantage is rapid action, the disadvantage is that they cause a hangover effect and therefore interfere with driving and with concentration even the next day. Antidepressants may be used for longer – several months if necessary because the modern ones do not cause drowsiness and so do not interfere with work or other physical activity (though they do have a long and increasing list of side-effects that you should discuss with your doctor).

Tranquillizers and antidepressants are not the answer to anxiety but they are part of the solution. They relieve anxiety enough for you to start to think constructively about the situation and to decide what form of further help might be appropriate. They are far preferable to drinking to excess or taking illicit drugs – those routes are solitary and empty and risk a spiral into addiction.

AND FINALLY

Do not forget about the basics of adequate sleep, good food and companionship.

Depression

Heroes do not get depressed – that is for wimps. Think again. Depression is widespread and often goes unrecognized. Men might prefer to call it 'exhaustion' or 'being a bit on edge' or 'nothing that a good drink and a night out with the mates won't cure'. These are all reasonable things to say during brief episodes of feeling low. But they are useless in dealing with more prolonged or severe depression and, in the case of drink, may even add to the problem.

WHAT IS DEPRESSION?

There are many disorders of mood of which depression is one example. By mood is meant the emotional state with which you deal with the world and within any one day this can swing between depression, optimism or feeling neutral. On the whole this is in response to events which have a psychological impact, such as criticism, success, conflict, pleasurable activities, upsetting events, family goings-on and work pressures. These are things to which we expect everyone to have some sort of emotional reaction – otherwise we call them cold or unfeeling or odd.

Psychological theories of mood and depression dominated thinking until fairly recently. Now it is increasingly accepted that depression can arise from disordered biochemistry within the brain. The brain is a mass of neurons (nerve cells) which communicate with each other using electrical signals. However, those signals cannot themselves jump the tiny gaps between nerve cells, called synapses. Jumping the gap involves a chemical process – the arrival of an electrical impulse stimulates the cell to release minute packets of chemical called a neurotransmitter. These drift across the gap to the next cell, where, on arrival, they stimulate an electrical discharge and so the signal gets carried forward.

These neurotransmitters are now believed to be deeply involved in mood and if they are decreased appear to cause depression. The ones most blamed are called serotonin or noradrenaline. Medical treatments work by boosting the levels of the neurotransmitters (see below).

COMMON SYMPTOMS OF DEPRESSION

These will vary from the very mild, which we all experience, to the more serious or even abnormal, which call for professional help.

- Lack of enjoyment of normally pleasurable activities with friends and family.
- Poor concentration.
- Disturbed sleep – lying there worrying about things.
- Feelings of sadness start to outweigh moments of enjoyment.
- You find it difficult to plan for a future which looks bleak or hopeless to you.

- You may experience various non-specific physical symptoms, such as headaches, tiredness, or not breathing deeply enough (see also Anxiety checklist on page 145).

These mild symptoms may or may not be obvious to others, unless you talk about the way you feel or unless their suspicions are alerted by a serious change from your usual behaviour.

The symptoms of more serious depression include:

- Seriously disturbed sleep and waking early in the morning in a state of agitation or gloom.
- Constant anxiety.
- Lack of libido (sexual drive).
- Loss of appetite.
- Inability to think in a purposeful way, because you are overwhelmed by anxiety or hopelessness.
- Turning to alcohol, drugs and other self-destructive behaviour, in an attempt to escape the constant mood of despair.
- Becoming convinced that you have a serious illness, despite reassurances.
- Crying, and thinking the worst.
- Contemplating suicide.

By the time you feel this bad, chances are that outsiders will have noticed something wrong and will be urging you to seek help.

WHAT TRIGGERS DEPRESSION?

Psychiatrists used to classify depression until recently as being either reactive (in response to life events) or endogenous (arising from within yourself). Though this is now felt to be an oversimplification, it is a helpful and easily understandable framework. Triggers to a reactive depression would include such major life events as bereavement, divorce, serious illness in yourself or close associates, money and job pressures. Triggers to endogenous depression include your basic personality and heredity interplaying with alcoholism, drugs and occasionally a physical illness such as an underactive thyroid gland.

WHAT'S ON OFFER FROM DOCTORS?

Doctors are likely to be your first port of call if you suspect depression or even if you just do not feel well in a vague way. They will want to know how you are feeling in detail; whether any triggers might explain your mood; whether you are drinking a lot and whether you have thought about suicide. All this is important in confirming the diagnosis and deciding the type and urgency of treatment.

You may well find it helpful simply to have explained to you how your array of symptoms all add up to depression. For milder cases this may be all the treatment required, other than psychological support.

Antidepressants

These have a bad reputation; this is because the older drugs had many side-effects. The most widely used were tricyclic antidepressants such as amitriptyline and dothiepin. That they do work is undisputed but the side-effects include drowsiness, a dry mouth, heart irregularities, blurred vision and constipation. In overdose (and this can be from just a few tablets) they make the heart beat erratically and are therefore dangerous. Tricyclics are still widely used because often sedation is needed at least in the early stages of treatment.

SSRIs

These are selective serotonin reuptake inhibitors. Their use is linked to the biochemical theories of depression and the role of neurotransmitters (see earlier). Serotonin is one of these neurotransmitters, lack of which is believed to underlie depression. SSRIs have become very widely used in recent years – brand names include Prozac and Seroxat. They are popular because they are much less likely to cause drowsiness and other side-effects, they do not affect concentration, they lift mood reliably and are safe in overdose. On the down side they may affect appetite (either increase or decrease), reduce libido, cause sweating or nausea and there is uncertainty as to their long-term safety.

Antidepressants – why take them?

Few thinking doctors would push antidepressants simply for the sake of it. There is a cunning plan. One of the problems with depression is to know where to start. How can treatment begin to help if the sufferer continues to see things through a black curtain of gloom? Antidepressants kick-start that process, by lifting a corner of the despair; you can begin to see that you do not have to feel the way you do, that treatment can help. Once your mood has lifted enough you are ready to respond to help offered by others, be that family, friends or counsellors. So though antidepressants are not the whole solution they are part of the answer.

For people who are suicidal, antidepressants are essential, given of course with care and supervision.

I'M NOT DEPRESSED

Not everyone can accept that they are depressed; it may just not fit in with how you see yourself and you may prefer to think you have some physical reason for your vague symptoms rather than accept that there is an emotional cause. Men especially consider that they are thick-skinned creatures, that emotional ups and down are simply part of life. They can tough it out. Well, maybe you can, but it can be a lonely road, risking disruption to family and work, and you may turn to alcohol or drugs to escape the pain. You cannot be forced to have treatment unless you are judged to be so depressed that the risk of suicide is high. In these circumstances people can be legally committed into a psychiatric hospital. And suicide is not a remote risk; in the UK about 4,500 people a year commit suicide. Of people who are severely depressed, 5–10 per cent eventually kill themselves.

HOW COUNSELLING AND PSYCHOTHERAPY HELP

Earlier we mentioned the theories of depression – reactive versus endogenous. Every case of depression has elements of both. Medication helps the biochemical side, but what about the psychological side? This is where the 'talking treatments' come in. For centuries, of course, there were no other options for depression but to talk about it. This reached a peak of development under the influence of Sigmund Freud and others who proposed theories of human behaviour. These theories make great reading but are increasingly believed to be founded on shaky experimental foundations. Nevertheless they are a way of getting behind simple emotions.

We now all take for granted the influence of early upbringing and frustrated desires, that what we say may be the opposite of what we mean and that events from long ago can influence later behaviour. Classical psychotherapy puts an emphasis on how sexual conflicts may underlie adult emotional states. This may be relevant in mild depressive states but it is unlikely in severe depression, where the biochemical model now prevails (see also Anxiety page 144).

All that talking...

This is a problem with classical psychotherapy; the argument goes that it's taken years for you to reach the state you are in, so how can you expect to escape without years in therapy? Few people have the time (or money) for extended therapy, which might easily continue for two years, which is why we now have brief psychotherapy and group therapy. These still need about six months of treatment, aimed at discovering how past experiences may be influencing your present moods. If you are lucky you will get this in one-to-one sessions with a psychotherapist; otherwise you will be in a group with others. Not everyone finds this to their taste, especially where there are problems of a deeply personal and therefore emotionally charged nature. Men particularly – never ones to express emotion readily anyway – can feel inhibited and awkward in a group.

Cognitive therapy

Simply put, cognitive therapy does not try to explain your moods; rather it tries to find ways of altering how you look at the things that are causing your moods. For example, you may be depressed at the fear of heart trouble and interpret perfectly natural variations in heart rhythm as meaning disease. Cognitive therapy, having identified such beliefs, would show you how your thinking is wrong – showing, for example, how activity influences your heart rhythm.

To benefit from 'talking therapies' you must be prepared to be frank and it helps to have insight into your psychological make-up. This comes less easily to men than to women (the wiring of the brain appears to be different). Men often feel silly, threatened, embarrassed, and are unused to expressing emotional worries. You may be concerned about confidentiality – that your therapy will get back to the boss. Be reassured that counselling takes place under strict conditions of confidentiality. Even where counselling is made available by your employer (as is increasingly the case), details should not be revealed without your consent.

WHAT COMPLEMENTARY PRACTITIONERS MIGHT OFFER

The range of therapies is set out under Anxiety, see page 144).

Self-help measures

It is difficult for people who are depressed to help themselves. Why bother, they say. Things are already so bad, they are bound to get worse. Your scope for action is at the onset of depression before it has taken hold and destroyed your motivation.

RECOGNIZE IT

A simple questionnaire that you can ask yourself is:

- Do you feel satisfied with your life?   (yes 0, no 1)
- Does your life feel empty?   (yes 1, no 0)
- Do you fear something bad will happen to you?   (yes 1, no 0)
- Do you feel happy most of the time?   (yes 0, no 1)

If you score two or more, you are quite possibly depressed. First you must accept your depression. Don't persist with any male macho stuff. Real men do get depressed and cannot cope. They may even cry! Then do something about it. Seek the forms of help outlined above.

REVIEW OBVIOUS STRESSES

Can you do anything about these; are they temporary or permanent; how serious are they really? Speak to someone about your feelings – your partner, doctor or friends. If they all agree you are depressed, it might just be that you are depressed!

I'm quitting tomorrow...

We all need little props to help us get through life, but sometimes props can gradually grow more and more important, until we find ourselves with a serious addiction or dependency. Addictions or dependencies can be a symptom of mental health problems, or a cause, or sometimes a mixture of both.

ADDICTIONS

In Part One we gave quit plans for those addicted to nicotine or alcohol. If either of these are problems for you, see pages 31 and 33).

Drug addiction, and addiction to other dangerous substances, as in glue sniffing, is a serious and often tragic problem which can ruin lives, careers and relationships – all the things we value. If you know you have a drug problem, or if you are worried that anyone you know or love might have a problem, seek professional help.

It is often obvious that someone is on drugs, but if it is not, then suspicion might be aroused if, for example, he or she shows wild and otherwise inexplicable mood swings, is sometimes uncharacteristically aggressive, is constantly short of money (possibly stealing to support a habit), and is evasive when questioned. Hard proof could include finding drugs-related equipment, or a supply of actual drugs.

If you need help, your GP is a good place to start; he or she will be able to put you in touch with specialized help groups. Or if you are a member of a religious faith, you could approach your religious leaders, as many religious organizations have volunteers who are trained to help in the battle against drugs.

The implication here is that the addiction is to illegal drugs, but prescription drugs, including tranquillizers, can also lead to addictions. Doctors are fully aware of this and carefully monitor their use. If you are concerned that you are coming to rely on any medication, talk to your doctor; there are ways you can gradually adjust your medication to wean you off possible dependency.

Addiction to gambling is also relatively common, and can have severely destructive effects on the victim's career, family life and personal relationships. Anecdotal evidence suggests the problem may have worsened since the advent of the National Lottery, which makes gambling so easy. If you very regularly gamble, especially if you risk far more than you can afford, if you steal to support a gambling habit, or if you feel compelled to gamble, then once again, seek professional advice. Or, if this describes someone you love, encourage them to seek help. Talk to your GP, or contact Gamblers Anonymous – the address is in the phone book. Again, if you are a member of a religious faith, your religious leaders may be able to help.

Almost anything can become the focus of addiction. Caffeine (found not only in coffee but also in tea and some fizzy drinks) is frequently cited. Sportsmen can also become addicted to the hormones the body produces during exercise and physical exertion. Many women claim to be addicted to chocolate (but men tend to think they just lack self-control). Many men claim to be addicted to sex (but women tend to think they just...)

If you suspect that you are coming to depend on a substance or, since recognizing addiction in yourself can be difficult, others keep trying to point out that you have a problem, then the following generalized quit plan might help. If not, talk to your GP.

Step 1: preparation
- Convince yourself you want to quit – half-hearted commitment will lead to failure.
- List the negative effects of your addiction (to give yourself good reasons to stop).
- Find some alternatives to replace the kick your addiction gives you.
- Mentally prepare yourself for a hard time when you first quit.

Step 2: giving up
- Give up all in one go – not gradually – and try to make a ceremony of giving up.
- Arrange some diversion for the first day you quit, to take your mind off any cravings.
- Reward yourself for each day you stay off your addiction.

Step 3: staying off
- Avoid trigger situations, which you know will tempt you to backslide.

- List the positive benefits of being habit free.
- Save the money you would have spent on your habit for a special treat.
- Continue exploring other sources for the buzz you used to get from whatever it was.

DEPENDENCIES

In recent years, there has been much discussion of dependencies and co-dependencies within relationships. This has often been in books and articles aimed at a female readership, but it is equally applicable to men, since men also get jealous, men also get compulsive, and men also get obsessive.

Dependency is not necessarily a bad thing. Most happy couples are dependent on each other, in the sense that they cannot do without each other...or they would not be couples. But dependency can get out of hand. One member of the partnership can become totally dependent on the other, who abuses that fact. Either partner can get obsessively jealous about the other, or even about the other's past. These can be thought of as unequal dependencies – one is dependent but the other is not.

In co-dependencies, on the other hand, suspicion, compulsion and obsession get all jumbled up to create misery and confusion within the context of a relationship so that neither partner feels able to end, or to leave – both are trapped by dependency.

Problems rooted in co-dependency can arise, in part, because members of a couple fail to communicate their needs, desires, hopes and anxieties to each other. If this is the case for you, see page 105, where we describe the issue of communication between men and women.

If the two of you have tried to resolve problems on your own but you feel that your relationship and your emotional life are still dominated by compulsive or obsessive feelings neither of you can control, and which you would both rather banish, then consider getting some professional help. Possibilities are from a relationship counsellor or therapist – the address for Relate is in the phone book.

REASONS TO BE CHEERFUL

The power of positive words and visual images has been known for thousands of years. Recently, formal techniques employing positive thinking have been harnessed. Businesses are increasingly encouraging staff to think for success, which is why there is such emphasis on mission statements, vision and values. Sportsmen place great emphasis on the inner game to maintain a positive mental attitude.

Positive thinking can have a tremendous impact on your mental health. If you are feeling down, why not try using affirmation or visualization to boost your mood?

AFFIRMATION

Affirmations are positive statements used to transform your mental outlook. They are tools for training the mind to think in constructive ways.

Affirmations should be:

- in the present tense: for example, 'I, Tom, am motivated and inspired', or 'I, Tom, am stress-free and relaxed';
- short and easy to remember;
- positively focused on the outcome you want, not negatively focused on your current problem: for example, 'I, Tom, am a confident and self-assured presenter', not 'I, Tom, am never nervous in business presentations'; or 'I, Tom, am always cool under pressure', not 'I, Tom, never lose my temper'.

Affirmations should incorporate your name (I, Tom...) They can be written down, spoken, or recorded on to tape. You can use them whenever or wherever you want – in the bath or on the bus. It might help if you try to repeat them silently to yourself in time to the rhythm of your breathing or, if you are walking, to the rhythm of your pace. You can introduce new ones as your circumstances change. Those which run counter to what is currently true for you are often the most helpful. For example, if Tom is subject to wild mood swings, affirming 'I, Tom, am calm and in control of my feelings' will strengthen and support his other efforts to deal with this problem.

VISUALIZATION

Visualization can be thought of as structured daydreaming to help you bring about the kind of mental states you would like to have. Start by trying to formulate a mental picture of the outcome you desire. For instance, if in your relationship you are made miserable and anxious by jealousy, you could picture yourself with your girlfriend at a party, with you looking on quite happily as she chats to another man. Then settle yourself somewhere quiet, warm and comfortable; minimize the possibility of distractions by unplugging the phone and asking other people to leave you undisturbed. If you use music in the background, make sure it is soothing. You can either sit or lie down, but if you choose to sit, make sure your back is well supported. Try to breathe regularly and deeply. Once you are settled, focus on the mental picture of your chosen outcome, and then just let your mind and imagination do the rest...

Programme for change

Part Three of this book has been about attaining and maintaining an even, calm and life-enhancing mental state, and about how you can manage the stresses and strains which are part of all our lives so that they do not permanently mar your happiness. We can all benefit from an increased awareness of what goes on in the mind – a point which women often accept more easily than men. There is nothing to be ashamed of in confronting issues concerned with mental health; use this programme for change as a first step to a new approach.

Step 1: identify what you want to change

Are you most concerned about unhealthy aggressiveness at work, chronic insecurity, managing a particular stress trigger, generalized anxiety, jealousy, obsessiveness...or what?

Only you can decide what you want to change. You are probably aware of the general area in which your problem lies, so start by trying to describe it in great detail, as accurately as you can. You need not share the result with anyone, but it might help if you could, since they might be able to help you clarify any potentially difficult issues. Even if you can only get as far as a description such as 'generalized anxiety', facing the problem is a first step to resolving it.

Let's take Don as an example. Don is sixty-three, married with three adult children, all living in London. He has always worked in retail, and is now manager of a department store in Leicester. When he retires, he and his wife Lil are considering moving back to their native Wales. He is deeply worried by the prospect of retirement: 'I'm afraid of all the time I'll have on my hands. I love Lil, but we're not used to spending all day together – how will that affect us? I want to return to Wales, but at the same time I want to stay put. I'll miss my job, and the responsibility – I'm worried I'll get bored with nothing to do all day.'

Don does not need to identify what to change, what he wants is a strategy for managing a major change – the change from fully paid-up member of the working population, to being a retired Senior Citizen.

Step 2: setting priorities

Once you have a description of your problem, you can set priorities for tackling it. Even a vague description can help. If your description is 'generalized anxiety', you could make it a priority to try to pin down the underlying cause, or seek professional help.

Don and Lil decided that their first priority was to make a final, definite decision about moving to Wales. Lil felt very strongly that she did want to return, to be near her sisters, and her nieces and nephews. Even after lengthy discussion, Don still felt ambivalent about any move, but as a couple they decided they would go back, and Don felt happy that the choice had been partly his – he had not been bulldozed into moving.

As a second priority, they decided that Don, who had few hobbies, should try to develop some outside interests now, two years before retirement, which would occupy and stimulate him afterwards.

Step 3: identify potential obstacles

If you identify obstacles you might face in overcoming mental health problems, you are less likely to be derailed by them.

Don felt that a big obstacle facing the success of his strategy to adopt outside interests was that he was now living in Leicester, but after retirement would be living in Wales. So if he got interested in anything locally, there would still be a big adjustment when he moved.

Lil was able to persuade him that most interests are transportable. OK, the friends he made through interests developed in Leicester would be left behind, but not his new skills. With some misgivings, he signed up for a photography course 'because I wanted to be able to take decent pictures of the grandchildren', and a computer course 'because my son kept telling me I'd get hooked on the Internet'. Six months later Don also signed up for an Open University degree in history – and thus fulfilled a long-standing ambition to pursue the higher education he'd missed out on as a younger man.

Step 4: set a timetable

How long are you prepared to give yourself, before you want to see results? Your timetable will, of course, depend on your individual aim, and timetables are often not as appropriate when dealing with depression, say, as they are in dealing with getting fit. Nevertheless, some sense of time-pressure can be helpful. If you decide to see a counsellor or therapist, and after three months you feel no better about any of your problems, it might be wise to reconsider your position.

Don and Lil had an inbuilt timescale of two years – two years in which they had a fantastic opportunity to plan for their future.

Step 5: review progress

In order to review progress, we suggest you keep a diary specifically for this purpose. Jot down anything which seems relevant to your chosen aim.

Just after he signed up for the OU degree, Don wrote: 'I feel so much happier about the prospect of retiring now. I'll be able to study in Wales, get out to the library, and so on. I've got plenty of interests to keep me busy, to stop me brooding, and keep me out from under Lil's feet!'

If you notice that progress is becoming stalled – for example, that your efforts to control generalized anxiety are not working – you will need to take immediate remedial action to prevent the situation deteriorating. Why not try making some affirmations, or visualizing success, as suggested above? You might also benefit from seeking professional advice. Your GP can always offer help.

Step 6: reward achievement

If you succeed in your aims, plan to give yourself a reward. If you overcome a major stress trigger, beat a dependency, bring your anger under control or whatever, you certainly deserve a treat.

Once Don and Lil had made the decision to move back to Wales, they celebrated with a meal at one of Leicester's top restaurants, and drank a bottle of Champagne – something they usually only did at weddings and christenings.

Only you can decide what would reward your achievement, but ideas might include buying yourself a relaxation tape, taking up a new hobby, joining a study group, taking a trip in a hot-air balloon, buying the gadget you been promising yourself...let your imagination run free, and choose anything to expand your mind.

If you fail in your aims, remember you did well to try, especially in the difficult area of mental health. For a man to accept that he may have a psychological problem is a big step – it rocks your self-image and threatens your self-esteem. However, it is no bad thing to be reminded that you are human after all. You can always try again.

PART FOUR
self-image
and
GROOMING

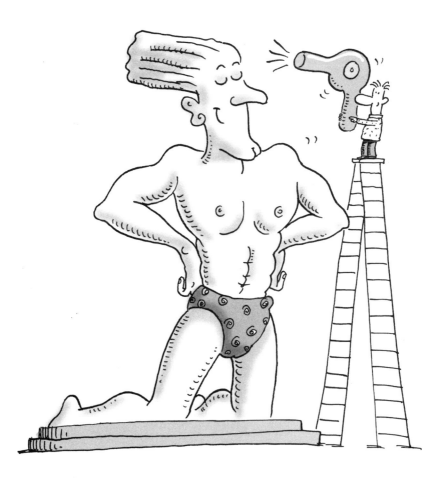

The basics

In this section, we examine those mainly physical things which have an important influence on how others react towards you. A constant theme is that the way others respond towards you influences the way you feel about yourself, which in turn communicates itself back to the outside world. This may not be a politically correct message – don't we all want to be loved for the deeply lovable creatures we feel ourselves to be? – but we hope you can cope with reality.

GROOMING
Sociable and sensitive grooming is about:

- maintaining an attractive exterior;
- protecting yourself from infection;
- clearing infection as soon as possible;
- not spreading infection to others.

Have you ever wondered why animals spend so much time grooming? All that licking of fur, scratching, peering and sniffing? Of course, many animals have thick pelts – parasites subsist on all living creatures and there is nowhere snugger for a bug to curl up than at the base of a warm layer of fur. Man, with a few exceptions, is a relatively hairless animal; even so, our skins, which are protection for our bodies, are prairies and hunting grounds for parasites. Furthermore any orifice offers a potential home to something that yearns after warmth.

Things that live on man
The world teems with micro-organisms. Bacteria are single-celled organisms capable of living and reproducing on their own. They are tiny; side by side you could fit from 1,000–10,000 to a centimetre. Many can move. They reach us through the air, in droplets coughed or sneezed out, through skin contact, when shaking hands, to anything more intimate. They are in the food we eat, the things we handle, the air we breathe. Here are some examples. Staphylococci cause many skin infections and boils, occasionally causing serious chest infections. E-coli is notorious for

giving a particularly unpleasant form of food poisoning, though usually it lives harmlessly in enormous quantities within our bowels. Haemophilus is responsible for meningitis and streptococci for throat infections.

Bacteria are at the root of the more common sexually transmitted diseases such as gonorrhoea (the gonococcus) and syphilis (the spirochete treponema pallidum). They also inhabit the mouth and will live under the nails and foreskin.

VIRUSES

These organisms, referred to by doctors to explain many minor illnesses, are unimaginably minute; 150,000 flu viruses side by side would measure just 1cm. Millions can inhabit a contaminated area yet remain invisible to the naked eye. If you have a cold, a single kiss can transfer more than the population of Britain. Viruses have no sex, but if they did they would be male, because all they consist of is a genetic code (DNA or RNA) within a protective coat and all they do is to invade other cells in order to take over their reproductive processes and produce more viruses. Illness results from the disruption to normal cell activity and the defensive actions of the body. Viruses are responsible for the common cold, flu, AIDS, and forms of throat and chest infection. Viruses do not respond to antibiotics, though there are just a few anti-viral drugs. The threat from commoner viruses can be controlled by vaccination, against polio, mumps and measles, for example.

FUNGUSES AND OTHER ORGANISMS

If the bacteria and viruses do not get you, then funguses will. A fungus is a strange creature, more like a co-operative organism than a single organism. Funguses grow by throwing out filaments which spread through the tissue they have invaded and then bud into new fertile bodies. Examples are candida and ringworm, and they commonly affect warm moist areas, such as under the foreskin, the groin, armpits and the scalp. You can recognize fungal infections because they cause a skin rash (usually slightly raised), are itchy and very slow growing.

If this makes the world sound a hazardous place for picking up infection – well, it is. Infections are generally more of a threat to health than things like heart disease or cancers – at least until middle age. In the developed world we are (or can be) protected by high standards of hygiene and the availability of antibiotics.

Cleanliness – doing it for yourself

One fundamental of grooming is to search for parasites and to keep our skins and hairy areas clean so they do not get there in the first place.

Cleanliness – doing it for others

Remaining well groomed ensures you are pleasant to be with, whatever your relationship – at work, with friends, or sexual partners. It is an important part of what is called your persona – a kind of summation of the whole you, that includes your physical and psychological qualities.

Personal hygiene

SCENTS AND STINKS

Among the bizarre products available through men's magazines, have you read about a spray cologne, which, it is claimed, will sexually attract women instantly? The idea is that the power of pheromones can be harnessed in a handy package to unlock women's wildest sexual desires.

The spray cologne might not have women throwing themselves at you, but it is true that scent is very important, both in the mating game, and in other spheres of life. Pheromones are powerful, highly scented substances that are secreted and released by animals, including man, to convey messages to others of the same species, especially those of the opposite sex. The natural smell of clean, fresh male, should be enough to drive women crazy – or the smell of clean fresh male supplemented by an aftershave or one of the conventional male colognes.

Your grandparents probably thought that only women with a nastier smell to hide wore scent, and men never did. But nowadays, men are happy to splash on beautifully packaged, heavily promoted blends of aromatic chemicals. Many perfumes targeted at men lean heavily towards woody, earthy scents or pungent spices, as these are deemed to enhance the natural odour of man – but whatever your taste, the range of scents available to you is nearly as wide as that for women, so you should be able to find something you like, should you want to.

So much for the smell of clean, fresh male of the perfumed or unperfumed variety. Now to something entirely different – the stinky, BO-ridden male. If you smell, you will drive people away – women, colleagues, people on the bus. It is basic advice, but make sure you wash regularly, use a deodorant and change your underwear at least daily. And washing regularly does not mean wiping your face with a flannel once a week. It means taking at least one bath or shower a day, plus showering or bathing after any particularly strenuous physical exertion at work or sport. Plus a quick wash-down before bed.

Apart from generalized BO, men frequently suffer from two other scent-related problems – smelly feet and bad breath.

SMELLY FEET

If you are a victim of smelly feet, this can be tackled with a variety of foot deodorizing sprays and powders, as well as shoe inserts. Check first whether you have athlete's foot, looking for cracked and itching skin between your toes. Your local pharmacist should be able to offer you advice. Take care of your feet with scrupulous daily washing; ensure that your socks, which should be changed at least daily, are of wool or cotton; and your shoes of leather, since these natural fibres enable your feet to breathe more easily than synthetics. If practical, try to go without either shoes or socks when you can. If you habitually wear trainers, throw them out before they are capable of walking off by themselves.

BAD BREATH

Bad breath has a variety of causes. Smoking is a common one – yet another good reason for giving up. If not removed by regular brushing, food debris around the teeth will start to rot, giving rise to noxious smells. Infection of the gums and rotten teeth can also lead to bad breath, as can sinusitis, tonsillitis and other minor local infections. More serious underlying disease, such as diabetes, can also sometimes be responsible for specific changes in the smell of breath.

Treating bad breath depends on the cause. Good dental hygiene – regular brushing and flossing – can deal with most cases. Rotten teeth may require extraction , so it is far better to make regular trips to the dentist before your teeth get into such a state of disrepair. Antiseptic mouthwashes should be used with caution as they can interfere with the normal bacterial content of the mouth and could encourage thrush. Depending on the extent of the problem, your GP might prescribe antibiotics to fight minor local infections. Although they do not provide a solution, in the short term bad breath can be masked by sucking on a variety of specially formulated lozenges, many containing peppermint. See also dental health (below).

If you torment yourself with the idea that your breath stinks, remember that those most concerned about bad breath do not usually have it, and those worst affected are usually oblivious to the problem.

DENTAL HEALTH

Quite apart from the link between bad breath and poor dental hygiene, it is important to maintain a clean mouth, to ensure that your smile and your teeth last as long as you do. Regular brushing after meals with a brush that is in good condition (not one with all the bristles chewed away) is necessary, but not sufficient. You also need to floss; this will help prevent your gums from receding – a major cause of tooth loss. Your dentist or dental hygienist will be able to advise if you need help choosing a toothbrush or floss – several types are available.

Many men are afraid to go to the dentist. Dentists know this, and do all they can to reduce any possible distress. The drills used to remove decayed parts of the teeth are now much quieter than they were in the past, so you will not have to cope with a terrifying high-pitched whine. Gas and air and local anaesthetics are widely used, and teeth may be extracted under general anaesthetic – especially wisdom teeth. If you are afraid of the dentist, hypnotherapy may prove helpful; considering the advantages of a full set of healthy teeth, it is surely worth a try.

HE'S GOT PERFECT SKIN...AND HAIR, AND NAILS...

If you suffer a particular skin problem, such as acne, or psoriasis, see page 66. Here we give advice on general skin care.

Women are told they should cleanse, tone and moisturize. The theory justifying this time-consuming and expensive palaver is fairly unclear – except to advertising executives, and the cosmetic companies who employ them. As we have already seen, men's skin is generally thicker than women's. Daily shaving reputedly helps the skin from sagging as the very act of shaving gives gentle massage to the underlying facial muscles. On the whole, men can be reassured that healthy skin does not depend on the use of the seductively packaged lotions and potions that interested parties are trying to persuade them to use, with increasing, and increasingly profitable success. However, there is value in doing the following:

- Use sun protection – keeping out of the sun is the biggest single favour you can do your skin. Always remember the golden rule: slip, slop, slap – slip on a shirt, slop on some protective lotion and slap on a hat. If you habitually engage in outdoor sports, especially extreme sports, include protective sun screens and blocks for your face with the rest of your kit. You need a very high factor block for your lips, nose and cheekbones.
- Eat a balanced diet – cutting down on alcohol, sugars and fatty foods.
- Get a good night's sleep.
- Do not smoke. Substances in cigarette smoke give the skins of heavy smokers a characteristic yellowish tinge and a leathery texture.
- Wash regularly with soap and water.
- Use a simple moisturizer, such as E45, available through any chemist's for minimal outlay.

Hair and nail care is also straightforward common sense. Wash your hair when it needs it, with any inexpensive shampoo. If you keep your hair short, you probably do not need to use a conditioner, although these are increasingly being sold to men. Since most men keep their nails short, you should have no difficulty keeping them clean.

Just as for skin, healthy hair and nails depend on eating a balanced diet. Vitamin supplements specially prepared to help you overcome short-term problems with your skin, hair or nails are widely available from pharmacies and health-food shops.

SNORING

This is a much-mocked yet underestimated source of friction between couples. While you awaken refreshed and energetic, your partner slinks around, bags under her eyes, having been kept awake by your efforts to rival a steam engine.

Snoring is caused by vibration of the soft palate (the back of the roof of the mouth) as you breathe. It is worse during deep sleep especially after a drinking session and if you sleep on your back, so experiment with different sleeping positions. You might even consider sleeping in a separate bed if you have been on the drink.

Though annoying, snoring is usually innocent. However, a warning combination is snoring plus daytime drowsiness. Or your partner might notice that you seem to stop breathing during the night. These symptoms occur typically in people who are overweight and especially in those who have a large collar size (say above 18in). If this is you, you may have sleep apnoea, a recently recognized condition where you really are chronically starved of oxygen. Specialized help is available from ear, nose and throat surgeons, who trim the soft palate in an operation. Speak to your doctor.

Self-image

The way we regard ourselves is what is known as self-image. It is how we would describe ourselves if asked to give a thumbnail picture. Self image is believed to evolve slowly during childhood and early adult life, as a result of our experiences and in particular how others react towards us. Poor experiences during those formative years give people a grossly distorted view of themselves, leading them to feel unattractive or unworthy. Conversely, a nurturing upbringing should leave you with a strong sense of your own self-worth.

Physical health is an important component to how we see ourselves. This happens in a number of ways. If you feel unwell, that colours how you see the world and feel about yourself. You get irritable, monosyllabic and grumpy (oh, you are that way any way?…feel free to skip this bit). Sick people naturally want to shut themselves away from others and this is almost certainly an ancient instinct to protect the general health of the herd – we are all still part of a 'herd').

Sick or diseased people look different; this will signal to others that there is a problem. You may have rash, a boil, dishevelled hair, be scratching, sneezing and so on. Just as you automatically tend to avoid people unwell in these ways, so people will steer clear of you.

You in turn look at yourself and see a sick bunny – your hair is lank, your skin blotchy and sallow. That does nothing for your self-image and will reduce your confidence. Of course, a cold soon goes, but things like recurrent boils, chronic cough or smelly feet will make people constantly wary of you.

IMAGE – YOU ARE WHAT YOU APPEAR TO BE

The concept of self-image is not new but has become of importance in our competitive world. So, however much you say you disagree, you may have to accept that the way you look signals the way you are. Image probably began as a reflection of physical health – good hair, teeth and skin. Things that others can take in at a glance, in the way that we all automatically size someone up on meeting them. By extension it comes to signal your psychological health. Dirty shoes, poorly pressed clothes say 'Hey, I think I'm a hot shot, but really I'm a slob'.

So you do your own thing and why should you care? Fine if your appearance is irrelevant to your job. But what if you are an advertising executive, a lawyer or a manager? Your down-at-heel shoes and frayed collar – others may doubt your ability to organize a campaign or a department if you cannot apply high standards to yourself. So, hero; you may rightly agree that a lot of image is boloney and conformity and congratulate yourself on being a free spirit – but then ask yourself this. Faced with two choices equal in other ways, would you take legal advice from someone who cannot match their shirt and tie? Or would you buy a computer from someone who cannot find a pencil to write down specifications, and then drops their papers on the floor?

IMAGE AND REALITY

You might think all this is nonsense – if image was everything, who would have taken Einstein seriously? OK, genius; you are saying that you are so essential to your job/partner/friends that they should overlook your bad breath and mud-encrusted shoes. You may be right and you may be the lovable maverick that people put up with for your other qualities. This can be a fragile hold on others' loyalties and you may find it counts for nothing when your abilities fail. Poor grooming and self-image will lose you that subconscious advantage in a competitive situation, when someone else, who does not know what a great guy you really are, has to make a quick decision on employing you or entrusting you with an important task. That is when your image may be crucial in getting the business.

RESPECT FOR OTHERS

Image and grooming are not just for yourself; they signal to others that you are prepared to go to some trouble to look good. They (and you) may well understand that this is not your free choice, that it is all part of the game of life, but they will appreciate that you have made the effort for them. When you dress up for an important interview, when you wash your hair or get a health problem sorted out, this says to others, 'I am not only doing this for myself. I am also doing this for you. I am still an individual and only human, but I want to do the best to make you feel more comfortable with me.'

So grooming is part of a politeness in society, and makes it a whole lot more pleasant to be around other people. It is up to you if you want to extend this to projecting an image of yourself that is very different from the reality. This is what is meant by power dressing: wearing clothes or doing things in order to say something about yourself that may not be part of your true self – wearing designer clothes says something about your taste and wallet; joining the right golf club says even more about your wallet and that you want to be part of a certain crowd (back to that 'herd' again). Just like an animal, you need to show allegiance to the herd by wearing the right insignias, sharing the same territory and drinking at the same watering hole. Deny it if you wish, but human psychology says that if you act the part, you are a long way towards being the part you act.

IMAGE IN A CYNICAL WORLD

We all know that we play many roles and that image and grooming are a type of game to assist role playing. It is possible to accept these rules in order to be part of a group and yet remain an individualistic hero. You do this by adopting those little touches of individuality which say 'Guys, we all know this is a joke, isn't it; and look, this is my way of saying I am still my own person'. Some people do this by wearing a gaudy tie, some by driving a special car. Just avoid socks which play 'Jingle Bells'...

Baldness

WHY DO MEN GO BALD?

Men share this problem with other apes. In the great majority of cases the hair loss is as a result of a combination of age and the effects of male hormones. Together these factors make the hair follicles go into a state of suspended animation. The pattern of male baldness is a very specific one. It starts with thinning of hair around the temples, spreading to include the crown of the head. Eventually you may be left with a few forlorn wisps on top and a fringe around the back.

Heredity plays an important part; if your father or brothers went bald before the age of forty, chances are that you will too.

THE NATURAL HISTORY OF HAIR

The average scalp contains 300,000 hairs, most of which are steadily growing from hair follicles. Every three years a follicle switches off and the hair growing from it is shed. After this the follicle remains in a state of rest for a while before starting up again. A sudden shock (which includes a severe illness) will cause more than usual numbers of follicles to switch off, with a resulting large loss of hair for a few weeks. The average daily hair loss is 50–300.

WHAT ELSE CAN CAUSE BALDNESS?

A few conditions lead to hair loss, though typically a localized hair loss rather than the male pattern baldness described above. Disease of the scalp, such as ringworm, causes the hairs to break off and those remaining hairs to look moth-eaten. This is treated with anti-fungal preparations available from your doctor.

Sudden hair loss may be due to an auto-immune condition (one where the body reacts against its own organs – in this case the hair follicles). The diagnosis is less likely in men than in women and requires blood tests to prove it. It may apply to you if you already have another auto-immune condition such as an overactive thyroid gland or pernicious anaemia. The treatment is not very effective; steroid lotions rubbed on to the scalp or injected into the scalp help some men.

Hairs are liable to be broken by trauma such as pulling or twisted by extreme hair styles and perms or unusual colourings. These cases will recover once the cause is removed.

BALDNESS IS NEXT TO HAIRINESS

The same male hormones involved in balding also stimulate hair growth elsewhere, hence the common association of early baldness and a hairy chest.

BALDNESS – A TURN ON?
Jo, a thirty-six-year-old accountant from Leeds, remembers, 'We used to have this chemistry teacher at school who was bald as a coot, but had the twinkliest eyes and a most compelling manner. I fancied him rotten and I've gone for bald men ever since – my husband is bald. As for Telly Savalas and Yul Brynner...'

WHAT CAN BE DONE

The treatment of baldness is the pursuit of the desirable via the dubious. Short of castration at an early age (a guaranteed preventative) 90 per cent of men are likely to experience hair loss eventually. The simplest medical treatments involve steroids rubbed or injected into the scalp. These do work, albeit only partially, but the effect wears off once the therapy finishes.

Minoxidil is a drug originally prescribed for treating high blood pressure which causes hair growth. It has to be used for several months before it even starts to have an effect, and the effect again wears off when the treatment stops. It is therefore an expensive and non-guaranteed option but does help some men.

Hair transplants take clumps of hair, with skin, from the back of the head (where you can spare it) and transplant them into the front. The surgery carries some risks of scarring and infection; however it does give good results and is an option to consider if you can put up with the cost of surgery and the embarrassment while you wait for the clumps of transplanted hair to grow.

WIGS AND HAIR PIECES

A skilfully woven wig is the only realistic option for many men. The best modern pieces look natural and are secure, depriving comics of a previous generation of a rich source of material.

BALDNESS – SOME COMMON THEORIES

Bald men are sexier

There is some truth in this, in that bald men do have slightly higher levels of male hormone, accounting for increased hair growth elsewhere. What has not been proven (at least not scientifically) is whether this generates an increased sex drive. This is an area calling out for research and is one where we suspect volunteers will not be a problem...

A warm scalp reduces hair loss

Again there is an element of truth in this. It is known that keeping the scalp warm will reduce the amount of hair lost during chemotherapy for cancer. It is not known whether this extends to men in normal health.

There are things to rub in which make hair grow

We have mentioned steroids and minoxidil. Other things suggested include malt extract, eggs, alcohol and apple cider vinegar. Conventional medicine would regard these as complete spoofs. Some 'hair restorers' may have acquired a reputation after being used by someone whose hair would have re-grown anyway (perhaps after serious illness). None stands up to scientific scrutiny, but then so few things in society do. They may have a psychological effect and this might also cause some hair growth.

> Emma, a thirty-three-year-old marketing executive, says, 'There's something about a smooth scalp that really gets me. My partner has a splendid head of hair, but he shaved it all off once as some sort of statement – he's in design and he thought it would be cool. I really loved it. I won't let him grow his hair back – the smoother the better for me.'

Excess body hair

Men themselves tend not to regard this as a problem, more a sign of their virility. But their partner's reactions may be less predictable. The ancient Egyptians despised it and shaved off all they could. But other ancient civilizations such as the Assyrians luxuriated in hair as a sign of manliness. And now? Some women loathe it while others love it.

> Jane, a twenty-four-year-old lawyer, reveals, 'I once had this boyfriend who had the hairiest shoulders. I used to stroke them and they felt just like an animal pelt – it really turned me on. My present partner has a hairy chest, but that's it. I wish he had a bit more hair for me to twist my fingers through.'

Man (here including women as well as men) are unusually hairless creatures. Their cousins the great apes and other primates show a healthy pelt and it is not at all well explained why human being are relatively hairless. In the great majority of cases, unusual hairiness is not caused by illness but is a family or racial feature. Southern Europeans and Mediterranean and Indian peoples tend to be hairier than northern Europeans. The Chinese and Japanese have little body hair.

Hairiness tends to go together with baldness, as they both depend on male hormones. So hairy men also tend to go bald earlier. The growth of hair on the chest and back depends on high levels of male hormones; this may be the origin of the belief that hairy men are more virile.

179

A FEW RARE CAUSES

Hair growth can be stimulated by steroids taken, for example, for severe asthma or rheumatoid arthritis, or phenytoin taken for epilepsy. Certain unusual tumours of the pituitary gland cause hairiness together with unusual growth (acromegaly), or an underactive thyroid gland. These cases apart, the rest are just in-built.

OTHER HAIRY BITS

While body hair is acceptable, less acceptable are hairy ears and noses. This is probably because it is more visible and less neat than other body hair. Hair in these places is an exaggeration of the normal and is never a feature of disease.

WHAT CAN BE DONE

If you have a lot of body hair, you really are stuck with it. Only an obsessive (or narcissistic) man would go to the trouble of shaving it off. In any case you would have to get help for shaving your back. Then you would have to cope with itching as the hair re-grows.

In theory you could have the hair follicles destroyed by electrolysis, using an electrical current to kill the follicle. While this could work for a few small areas, it is a forlorn task for generalized body hair.

Removal with wax hardly bears thinking about. There are depilatory creams, which dissolve hair. Again, the effort required to remove a significant amount of hair hardly seems worth the effort.

DOES HAIRINESS MATTER?

Only for your own body image. Hairy men are not at any greater risk of skin trouble as a rule. Occasionally you may get boils at the root of hairs where they get rubbed or traumatized – on the face, buttocks and thighs. These can be treated with antibiotic creams or by taking antibiotics orally.

Cosmetic surgery – the hype and the reality

According to the hype, cosmetic surgery is a kind of insurance, enabling older men to turn back the clock and thus, in our youth-obsessed culture, resist competition from their more youthful rivals in both professional and personal spheres. In reality, of course, nothing puts back the clock – have a facelift, and ageing starts up again the minute the surgeon puts down his knife. A cheaper method of delaying the effects of ageing is to stay out of the sun.

In the USA 25 per cent of cosmetic surgery patients are men. Whereas ten years ago the majority of men enquiring about cosmetic surgery were interested in hair transplants, today men request information on facelifts, nose jobs, ear reduction and more. Common reasons for taking this route include:

- the hope of winning a job promotion, or a rise;
- the hope of finding a new mate, following divorce;
- boosting general self-image;
- enhancing physical fitness.

In the UK, it is probably fair to say that only our leading politicians are as image obsessed as the Americans. Nevertheless, it is probably also fair to say that more and more British men are willing to consider cosmetic surgery. If you fall into this group, you need to be clear on a few points before you even talk to a specialist.

- Can you clearly describe your desired outcome from surgery? If not, wait until you are sure about what you are trying to achieve.
- Is someone else pressuring you to have surgery? If so, resist.
- Are you reasonably happy and stress free? If not, bear in mind that your emotional state is perhaps not the best in which to evaluate the pros and cons of surgery.
- Do you hope that surgery will revolutionize your emotional, social or professional life? If this is your hope, it is a false one.

If you do opt for strictly cosmetic surgery, only in rare instances will this be available on the NHS. Nevertheless, it is worth discussing your plans with your GP before booking a consultation, as he or she will be able to give you general advice, and recommend a reputable surgeon. If you approach private practitioners direct, always ask how long they have been in practice, and which procedures they perform most often – you do not want surgery carried out by someone who only rarely performs the operation you require.

COMMON PROCEDURES

Only the most common cosmetic operations are listed below. Without being alarmist, it is worth pointing out that like all surgery these operations carry varying degrees of risk. Ask yourself whether the risks are worth it for purely cosmetic benefit.

Nose job

WHAT IS IT?

A nose job (rhinoplasty) alters the structure of the nose either to correct a deformity, perhaps caused by a sporting injury, or to improve the appearance of a healthy nose. We perceive a balanced face as attractive. A nose that is 'too large' can make the face seem unbalanced, and hence unattractive – at least in the eyes of its owner, who hopes surgery can provide him with a natural-looking, masculine nose, in proportion with the rest of his face.

HOW IS IT DONE?

The surgery is usually done under local anaesthetic. Incisions are made inside the nose, so there should be no visible scarring. These incisions uncover the wall of cartilage and bone which divides the nose into two cavities. The cartilage is reshaped, and bone is either removed, or supplemented with grafts from elsewhere in the body.

WHAT WILL I LOOK LIKE AFTER SURGERY?

You will be required to wear a splint on your nose for about five days. Packing will be put in your nose for the first few days, so you have to breathe through your mouth. There will be swelling and bruising around your eyes, and possibly over your cheeks, for about a week after surgery.

PITFALLS

Your skin type and age will greatly affect the results of this type of surgery. Thin, dry skin shrinks and reveals the modelling of the nasal bone and cartilage after surgery. Thicker, oily skin does not shrink back so well. Older skin will not shrink back after surgery as well as younger skin, so beyond middle age results are unlikely to be spectacular.

IS IT AVAILABLE ON THE NHS?
Only if there is a clear medical reason for surgery , such as if you find it difficult to breathe through your nose.

Ear surgery
WHAT IS IT?
About 90 per cent of ear growth is reached by the age of five, so unusual prominence is more noticeable in children than in adults. Girls can usually hide conspicuous ears under their hair, but boys frequently cannot. Young boys are often teased for having ugly or bat-like ears. Ear surgery (otoplasty) is most frequently performed on this group, but adults can also have protruding ears fixed.

HOW IS IT DONE?
Procedures vary, depending on the precise cause of the problem, the angle between the ears and the head, etc. But all incisions are made on the back of the ear, and cannot be seen after surgery. Children are usually admitted to hospital the day before their operation, and go home the following morning. A light general anaesthetic is used. Adults can often have the procedure done on an outpatient basis, with local anaesthetic.

WHAT WILL I LOOK LIKE AFTER SURGERY?
For about a week after surgery you must wear a turban-like dressing to make sleeping more comfortable and to protect your ears during healing. Following surgery, it may be necessary to take painkillers for a couple of days, and although you can wash your face, showers must be avoided for about week.

PITFALLS
The risks are low; bleeding and infection are rare.

IS IT AVAILABLE ON THE NHS?
Yes for children, probably not for adults.

The eyelift
WHAT IS IT?
The eyes, the windows on our souls, are our most expressive features. They are also, unfortunately, where age shows itself the earliest. In some unlucky men, especially those who have had a lot of exposure to sun, bags or circles around the eyes may appear in the thirties. The eyelift (blepharoplasty) is one of the easiest cosmetic operations, and can have significant results. An eyelift will not make you look twenty years younger, but it can given you a refreshed look, adding a note of vitality that may have been lost over the years.

HOW IS IT DONE?
The skin of the eyelids is very thin, so the surplus can easily be picked up and cut off. Usually, both upper and lower lids are operated on, but they can be done independently. The incision for the removal of skin above the eye is made in the crease of the eyelid, that for the removal of skin below the eye is made just below the lower lashes. Neither incision should leave scarring. The operation can be done on an outpatient basis, under local anaesthetic. Painkillers are usually prescribed afterwards.

WHAT WILL I LOOK LIKE AFTER SURGERY?
Bandages are usually positioned, but are not essential. When the eyes are exposed, ice compresses need to be applied frequently during the first thirty-six hours. For several days after surgery, you will look as if you have been in a fight – your eyes will be puffy, swollen and bruised. You will be able to return to work after a few days, but might feel like wearing dark glasses until the swelling and bruising subside.

PITFALLS
Risks are minimal – in very rare cases, excessive skin may be removed, so that the eyes cannot close comfortably.

IS IT AVAILABLE ON THE NHS?
Unlikely.

The facelift

WHAT IS IT?

A facelift removes sagging folds of skin on the cheeks, chin and neck. It cannot get rid of fine lines and hatch marks caused by sun damage. Women usually ask for facelifts in their fifties, men tend to wait until their sixties. This is partly because men have naturally thicker skin than women, which together with daily shaving helps prevent sagging to a certain degree.

HOW IS IT DONE?

In a facelift, incisions are made in the skin, which is then freed and pulled backwards and upwards to tighten it in various directions. Because men and women have differing patterns of hair growth, facelifts are performed slightly differently in the two sexes. In men, no incision is made in the scalp above the ears because future hair loss could reveal such scars. The naturally hairless area between the ear and the sideburn must also be preserved, and the natural hairline must be maintained at the back of the neck, since men usually keep their hair shorter than women. The facelift incision begins at the front of the sideburn and goes back into the hair and across the back of the head, parallel to the natural hairline. The operation is usually done under a general anaesthetic, but a local is also possible.

WHAT WILL I LOOK LIKE AFTER SURGERY?

Immediately following surgery, you will look quite a fright, with extensive swelling and bruising. For a couple of days, you might even have to live with surgical drains to prevent blood clots forming under your recently freed skin. Sometimes one side of the face heals more quickly than the other, so results look uneven – but this is thankfully a temporary effect.

PITFALLS

The freeing of the skin is extensive, and must be carried almost to the eye, and close to the mouth. There are very slight risks of damage to the nerves which supply the facial muscles, leading to facial paralysis. As already mentioned, there is also a slight risk of blood clot formation under the freed skin; this can cause various problems, including excessive scar formation.

IS IT AVAILABLE ON THE NHS?
Unlikely, except where a previous paralysis has affected the face.

OTHER WAYS TO CHANGE YOUR APPEARANCE

In addition to the cosmetic surgical procedures listed above, a variety of other means of changing your appearance are also available including:

- Tattoo removal – a boon if you have 'Rosie' tattooed on your biceps and your current girlfriend is called Sue, or if the results of a youthful indulgence in body art are deemed inappropriate for your current position at the merchant bank.
- Cosmetic dentistry to improve badly positioned teeth. Ask your dentist if you are interested in this option.
- Micro- or laser-surgery to correct short sight and prevent the need either for glasses, or contact lenses, with all their attendant hassle. Some opticians, especially in London, have block bookings with private consultants, which renders this procedure affordable.

There are also plenty of dodgier means of improving bodily defects. Many men's magazines carry adverts for procedures, techniques and products – creams, lotions, pads, pumps, implants and electronic stimulators, etc., which, it is claimed, can eliminate almost any physical imperfection. For example:

- Penis enlargement ('you too can go from minuscule to mammoth and have erect measurements of up to twelve inches').
- Hair and hair follicle transplants ('this procedure defies detection').
- Chest expansion and reduction, including pectoral implants ('build rock-hard muscles without exercise, fast').
- Abdominal sculpting ('an amazing new way to have that rippled muscle effect, for a lean hard look').
- Buttock sculpting ('eye-catching buttocks, instantly').
- Leg sculpting ('electrical impulses work your muscles safely and effortlessly').

If you are tempted by any of the products offering penis enlargement because you have difficulties achieving or maintaining an erection, then talk your worries over with your GP, as there are now safe effective NHS treatments (see page 100).

If you are tempted by any of the other instant roads to physical perfection, remember:

- perfection is not achievable;
- most safe and permanently effective methods of changing your shape do mean effort – they require you to develop a challenging exercise programme, and to follow a decent diet;
- changing the shape of your buttocks, or whatever, might cause a few women to ogle you, but it will not revolutionize your emotional, social or professional life;
- things can go wrong, leading to scarring, unnatural appearance and infection. If you do opt for any type of cosmetic surgery, always choose a reputable clinic or follow your doctor's recommendation.

Check out your voice

One very important, but often neglected aspect of self-presentation is the voice. The first things people notice about you are your eyes and your voice, and they use these as clues to make instant judgements. Politicians, businessmen and others in the public arena know this, and are often willing to spend time and money on voice training to help them change their images. Famously, both Margaret Thatcher and the Queen modulated their voices and brought them down in pitch. Pitch is important because lower-pitched voices sound soothing and authoritative, while high-pitched voices sound strident and bossy. Men have a natural advantage over women in this respect, but if you do worry that you sound squeaky, hum down the scale and pitch your voice at a level where you are not straining, but which you can easily maintain for short lengths of time.

If you have to make a speech, perhaps at a wedding or during a business presentation, practise what you are going to say in front of a mirror beforehand. This will help you judge what sort of impression you are likely to make (you can also practise ordinary conversations in this way). On the big day, loosen your voice to help you sound relaxed and at ease. If you can find some privacy, sing up and down the scale before you go public. If not, you can at least nip into the nearest toilet and loosen your jaw by moving it from side to side, making chewing motions and stretching your facial muscles in exaggerated smiles and yawns.

Body language is also part of the overall impression. Always look your audience in the eye, though without staring. If you refuse to look at people directly, by looking up or down or constantly shifting your gaze, it suggests you are hiding something, or are being economical with the truth. Remember though that outright staring is usually threatening, and makes others uncomfortable. When speaking, do not stand like a piece of wood; use your hands to illustrate points, and make expansive, inclusive gestures with your arms. Never waggle your forefinger, as this is aggressive. Folding your arms shuts people out – you are sending the message that you are unapproachable. Smile when speaking – smiling warms and enriches the voice. Show enthusiasm, even if this is an act – enthusiasm gets people's attention.

It is, of course, important to use language that is appropriate to the occasion. In social settings, don't use technical, work-related jargon as other people may fail to understand you and dismiss you as a geek or a show-off. We all have our favourite words and phrases; try to ensure you don't use your pet phrases so often they become irritating –I mean, you might be over the moon that, I mean, the sales force is, like, all singing from the same song sheet, but, like, the rest of us are bored to tears and, like, have murder in our hearts at this moment in time.

Here are some more specific pointers on using the voice to help you project a confident, impressive image. Use them judiciously, and people will listen when you speak, even if what you are actually saying is pure flannel.

- Slow down – if you speak too quickly, it suggests nervousness, which can place you at a disadvantage when answering questions, undertaking negotiations, inviting a woman to go to bed with you, etc.
- Vary your voice, i.e. vary the pitch, tone, speed and inflection – when we are nervous our voices flatten out, so we sound boring.

If you sound boring, you can be sure you are boring your audience, and you will quickly lose everyone's attention.

- Keep your voice up at the end of sentences. This will help you sound positive; if you let your voice drop, you will sound downbeat. If you do not want to discuss an issue, it is still important to sound positive. Answer difficult questions very briefly – assertively, but not aggressively – and finish on a rising, positive note (listen out for this trick next time you hear a politician being interviewed).

- Think about how long you have been speaking. When answering questions, do not be too brusque, but do not expand too much either. Aim to speak for roughly twenty seconds – this is a lot of words. Remember this advice next time you are at a dinner party and the smile on the face of the woman sitting next to you starts to look a little strained. (Dylan Thomas put this well when he wrote: 'Somebody's boring me. I think it's me.')

- Do not speak too loudly. Speaking too loudly causes embarrassment to those in your party who do not like their conversations to be overheard; it is also intrusive on other people's privacy. You might be interested in what you are saying, but the rest of the restaurant almost certainly is not. In large groups, do not shout, but project – put power into your voice.

If you want an honest opinion about the image you project both in general conversation and in more formal settings, ask a trusted friend to give you an opinion and to point out any minor idiosyncrasies.

Voice training is widely available in large companies as part of courses on making presentations, or as part of media training, which teaches executives who might be in the firing line how to cope with media interest should a crisis break out in their organization. If you are interested in this sort of professionally focused advice, you will find speech and language therapists in the Yellow Pages (try to get recommendations). If you are simply interested as an individual with general social concerns, then make enquiries in the drama and music (singing) departments of your local college of Higher Education, as suitable courses will probably be on offer.

Programme for change

Part Four of this book has been about the image you project, and how you can use image to enhance different areas of your life, especially your relationship and career prospects, both now and in the future. Although it is often treated as a female domain, there is nothing feminine in learning to manipulate the image you project to the world. It is an important skill, as leading politicians know only too well – the more aware you become of the image you project, the more aware you will become of how others are using image to manipulate you. Use this programme for change as a first step to a new you – but remember that changing the way you appear to the world cannot solve any fundamental problems in your life.

Step 1: identify what you want to change

Which elements of your current image do you most want to change? Are you most concerned about getting your body into shape? Getting to grips with BO? Protecting your skin from the weather? Softening your aggressive tone of voice, or what?

Only you can decide what you want to change. Start by drawing up a wish list of targets for change. Let's take Charlie as an example. Charlie is in his early twenties, has just completed a degree in English at Birmingham and is about to start work as an advertising trainee in London. He is single and describes his image as 'non-existent'. This is a state of affairs he wants to change, in accordance with all the other major changes taking place in his life.

Charlie's wish list of targets for change includes: 'do something about my hair; get some new clothes; get some new clothes; get some new clothes'.

Step 2: set priorities

Setting priorities obviously was not a problem for Charlie – he definitely wanted some new clothes. But for many people, setting priorities would be harder. If this applies to you, ponder your wish-list for a few days; you are not in a race to change your life. Then choose just one target – one area you would like to change, which you feel would have the greatest impact on your image. Perhaps this is to do with your personal hygiene routine – or lack of it – or something connected with your body language. Once you have achieved change in this key area, and reaped the benefits, you can come back to your other priorities.

Step 3: identify potential obstacles

If you identify potential problems in advance, you are less likely to be derailed by them.

The main obstacle preventing Charlie from getting some new clothes was his severe lack of funds. He was lucky in that his parents generously gave him the money to buy two suits, a couple of shirts, some ties and some new shoes, so he did not have to worry about his business wardrobe. But he imagined he had no casual clothes, or at least none which he felt to be suitable for his new life in London. He was wrong about this. His sister was roped in to help him overhaul his wardrobe, and she persuaded him to throw away many really tatty, filthy T-shirts, jeans, sweaters and other items. He was left with a core of quite presentable clothes, which could form the basis of his casual wardrobe for a few weeks, or months if necessary. 'I was quite surprised to find what I did have, I'd forgotten half of my stuff. My sister was quite a bully about what I could and couldn't keep, and I'm left with a few good things which do look OK together. She's kindly promised to come on a shopping trip with me, when I've got the money to get some new stuff.'

Step 4: set a timetable

How long are you prepared to give yourself before you want to see results? Your timetable will, of course, depend on your individual aim, and when it comes to self-image and grooming, results can be surprisingly quick. Charlie's shopping trips for new suits took up a couple of afternoons, and he and his sister spent another day going through his wardrobe. A new haircut takes a matter of minutes. Losing a beer belly will obviously take longer, but you must have some sense of time pressure, otherwise your project is likely to drift.

Step 5: review progress

In order to review progress, and monitor the image you are presenting to the world, we suggest you keep a diary specifically for this purpose. Note down what image you think you are projecting, and also how you feel about it. That way if you start to feel unhappy with your image, you can take immediate remedial action. After he started work, Charlie wrote: 'Wearing a suit makes me think I look like I know what I'm doing, even if I don't – it gives me confidence.' You could also note down any insights you gain about how other people are using image to influence you.

Step 6: reward achievement

If you succeed in modifying your image, give yourself a reward. Charlie decided that his reward would be to buy a new winter coat – when he could afford it. Other ideas might include drinking at a bar where you previously felt out of place, joining the gym now you can match pectoral to pectoral, buying a book or video on body language, etc. Let your imagination run free, and enjoy yourself.

If you fail to change your image, never mind. It took you decades to acquire it; it may take several attempts and much soul-searching to change it. Trying to alter one's image forces all thinking males to question what they want to represent in life. But though you may be undecided about this, do not overlook the fundamentals of basic hygiene and maintaining a confident expression. These are never a waste of time.

PART FIVE
the
HEALTH
hero

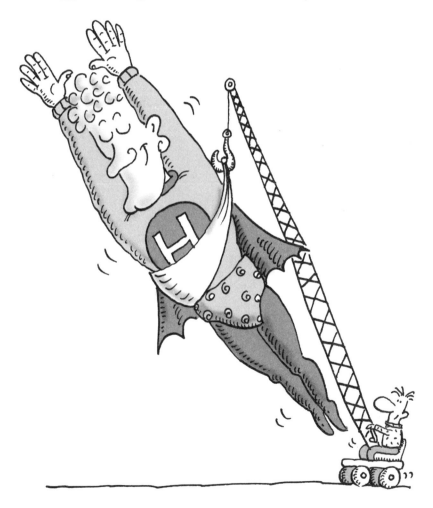

Advantages of being a health hero

In Part One we asked, 'Who are the health heroes?' and answered that becoming a hero means being willing to change, to put aside old ways of thinking and to open up to ever-expanding networks of possibilities. This whole book has focused on bringing about change in four key areas of life – physical, mental, sexual and perceptual (for what is image, if it is not to do with perception?) To be prepared to change means having the basic heroic qualities of vision and versatility. If you have worked through our programmes for change, you must have those qualities in abundance and deserve congratulations. Now it is time to consider the rewards your heroic status will bring you in terms of total fitness of mind and body, and of achievement – i.e. of well-being. We now focus on ten advantages, but you will discover that there are also many others.

INTEGRITY

This above all: to thine own self be true,
And it must follow, as the night the day,
Thou canst not then be false to any man.
Shakespeare

The health hero might say: 'I'd rather think and speak for myself and have no audience, than speak and think for an audience and have no self.'

Integrity? In this modern world of image, slickness and opportunism? It might seem hopelessly outdated. Yet it is a paradox that the more uncertain the world, the more important it is to have standards in order to resist relentless buffeting by outside pressures. You can tell this is not an outlandish thought by browsing through any book store. There you will find a huge range of titles on self-help and reaching happiness that are there because so many people feel a need for guidance on how to lead their lives. It may be for just such reasons that you are reading this book. Everyone at some time has to feel they can justify the way they are and be prepared to face an audit, as it were, of the way they live.

For some people a religious faith satisfies this need for rules by setting standards against which to measure yourself. A problem with religious standards is to find standards that are relevant to the modern world. For Christians, the Ten Commandments are a pretty good starting point, but nevertheless it can be difficult to relate religious precepts to modern demands.

Many people work out their own standards, drawing on examples which feel right for themselves, gradually accumulating rules for their behaviour which we recognize as integrity. Integrity begins as a quality personal to yourself, though it will communicate itself to others eventually. You are more likely to know when you lack integrity rather than when you have it. It is that curiously deflated feeling that comes after you have sold some equipment that you know is not really right for your client's needs, a feeling which lasts longer than the satisfaction you had felt at closing the deal. Or it is the gnawing knowledge that you have fitted some electrical cabling which your client will never see but which you know you have botched. There is no objective reason why you should take trouble to do a first-class job except for that internal auditor called conscience whose pencil hovers over a tick or a cross.

Such matters do have a habit of getting known to a wider audience, which is when you acquire a reputation for integrity, or otherwise. 'Give the job to so and so,' your colleagues may say. 'He'll get it done.' 'Jim? He can be a bit awkward but you don't have to keep watching him and the customers don't complain.' Other words people might use are 'reliable', 'conscientious' and 'his own man'.

Integrity can be an awkward virtue; you are not inclined to compromise and that nagging auditor may stand between you and a quick, dubious opportunity. Nor can any man possibly maintain consistent integrity in all his dealings; that will lead to feeling guilt and dissatisfaction. Nor can integrity be a goal in itself; that way you may end up as a self-righteous prig and still not too happy with yourself.

Integrity may be seen as unrealistic weakness in a demanding world, whereas it is completely the opposite. To stand firm when you are answerable to no one but yourself, to meet standards imposed by nothing other than your conscience – this is strength indeed.

STAMINA

Constant dripping wears away the stone.
Proverb

The health hero might say: 'My life is so packed, I haven't got time to be tired.'

It is all very well to know where you are going and how you are going to get there, but suppose you just get tired on the way? Stamina means staying power, both mental and physical. The physical side is easier to train up – this book includes programmes to help you do so. Be sure you feel good about your body, and get regular exercise as described. Especially get help for aches and pains – these are minor in themselves but they drain your mental strength. For much of the time physical fitness lies in reserve; it is when you are up against demands that you will be glad to know your body has the strength to keep going for as long as your mind can.

Mental stamina is harder to control and there is probably a large inborn element to it; some people are just naturally active, need little rest and have apparently endless energy. Others have to pace themselves and can work only in short bursts. So the first step is to know yourself through the techniques covered in Part Three. By now you should know something about how to clear your mind, and how to recognize and deal with the anxieties, doubts and depressions that affect all thinking people.

Remember some tricks for enhancing stamina in whatever area it may be – sport, work or relationships.

- Break your large tasks down into manageable targets, then set yourself a goal.
- Concentrate on finishing each segment rather than worrying about the whole.
- Reward yourself for each successful completed stage – this can be a mental pat on the back as much as a physical treat.
- Monitor your performance and rest once it is clear that you have outreached your stamina, before you are carried off the pitch.

Stamina is not an end in itself, but the means to an end. Keeping going simply for the sake of doing so is just activity masquerading as achievement, something which you as a thinking person are too self-aware to be fooled into.

LONGEVITY

Death closes all: but something ere the end,
Some work of noble note, may yet be done,
Not unbecoming men that strove with gods.
Tennyson

The health hero might say: 'I'll never lose my zest for life. People sometimes ask, "Who'd want to live to be a hundred?" Me, please.'

Now that the killer diseases of childhood are so rare, a long life is within everyone's reach. Why squander that possibility? Throughout this book there are hints on building and maintaining a healthy lifestyle – and, just as important, taking notice of those early-warning signs which men are so often inclined to ignore. As we hope you will agree, the necessary changes to diet and activity are not difficult nor unrealistic, whatever the other demands on you.

It remains true that the big influences on your life expectancy are unfortunately pre-set – your parents and their parents will have passed on a genetic legacy that will largely determine how long you will live and what diseases you are prone to. But just because it is genetic does not make this legacy unalterable. As an example, height is another genetically determined factor, yet average height has steadily increased over the last hundred years thanks to good nutrition. There are limits to your final height but good care allows you to reach your maximum potential.

Longevity is not just your business, it matters to others, too. A life ending unnecessarily early affects your relatives and loved ones. As a health hero, you will have seen how to be in charge of your body, determined to control those aspects of life that you can influence – diet, safety, exercise, and avoiding the risks posed by alcohol and cigarettes.

A long life is a life full of opportunity; there are new horizons, physical as well as mental, that you can sample whatever your age. It seems a waste to be living in one of the most diverse societies the world has ever known and not to experiment with the menu on offer – travel, hobbies, sports plus seeing, doing, commenting on and trying out numerous possibilities.

And what about clinging on to life, when quality has gone? There are a few individuals who face this unpleasant fate, but the numbers are relatively small. Though you cannot avoid ageing we hope we have shown you how to preserve the best of what you have. Most readers can look forward with reasonable confidence to living well into their seventies and eighties, and should regard every day as furthering that long opportunity.

Ah well, perhaps one has to be very old before one learns how to be amused rather than shocked.
Pearl Buck

SENSITIVITY

A healthy male adult bore consumes each year one and a half times his own weight in other people's patience.
John Updike

The health hero might say: 'I aim to be sensitive to other people's deeper needs and emotions, and not just to the effect I myself am having on them.'

There is a notion that sensitivity is only for wimps and that real men do not cry. Such an attitude will leave you bewildered and uncertain when strong wimpish emotions sweep across your progress through life. Or when people react in a puzzled and hurt way because you have failed to recognize their unspoken emotions. We hope to have opened your eyes to the richness and desirability of other ways of feeling.

Of course, it is possible to progress through work, sport and love while adhering to a philosophy of 'don't hear, don't care'. Such people may be admired for a while for the bottom line of what they achieve and the results they bring in. There is a place for insensitivity in all our lives or we risk being rendered paralysed for fear of how others may be affected by our actions. And it is often a selfish world; we demonstrate altruism in few and controlled ways. But imagine yourself at the receiving end of constant insensitivity and think of the pain, misery and ultimate destruction of relationships that such constant indifference does to others.

We hope we have shown that sensitivity to others works in your best interests – when you understand others' emotions you are better placed to influence their behaviour. Since everyone's favourite subject is themselves, you need display only a little sensitivity in order to get people to open up.

Be prepared for a few surprises. If people think you care about them, they will trust you and reveal aspects of their personalities that might otherwise have remained hidden. Regard this as power if you like, or (better and less cynically) as a meaningful relationship. Try to keep such cynicism for the day job.

Men find it difficult to keep up the introspection that can be part of sensitivity; you are likely to cut short revelations about your inner self when they threaten to become too emotionally engaging – or when the alcohol wears off. Women, as you may have noticed, regard sensitivity to emotions not as a bolt-on extra but as a necessary aspect of relating to others. Your children will expect you to be sensitive to their emotional needs no matter how opaque that seems even to themselves. Avoiding sensitivity may lead to bewildered and awkward relationships with your children as they grow older.

It is possible to lead life on just a few emotions – anger, excitement, lust and drowsiness do for some people; but as a health hero you could move into the richer worlds of self-knowledge and of trying to know others. If you wish to achieve lasting and satisfying relationships, spread some sensitivity around. You are more likely to keep your partner, impress your boss and startle your colleagues.

DESIRABILITY

O lyric Love, half angel and half bird
And all a wonder and a wild desire
Robert Browning

The health hero might say: 'I know I'm a walking streak of sex, and it's great.'

It is not only Greek gods and goddesses that fall in love; all the rest of us Johns and Janes do too. It follows that there must be more to male sex appeal than having a Greek nose and tight buttocks. Given that most of us are ordinary, we all have to make the most of what we have. Therefore it is all the more important to keep your body in best possible shape and show that it is in good shape, too. This is why your skin, hair and nails are important. In signalling to others that the visible goods are in order, you imply that the hidden bits are also likely to be. We have given guidance on achieving this.

So your muscles are taut, your skin is supple, your eyes are shiny and your hair is clean. Will the women come to you in droves? Yes they will; there's no point in denying it, attractiveness does what it says – attracts. But there is another aspect to your desirability – your personality; that is to say your attitudes, opinions, habits and all those facets of your behaviour which make you uniquely you. These are in many ways more important for long-term relationships; there is an interplay with your physical appearance – if you feel good about how you look, you will feel better and more confident about who you are. This is all to do with your self-image, which is both a strength and a source of strength.

Power and success will also make you desirable, and this is not just through a cynical attraction to your money. There is a desirability that emanates from attractive people who know that they are successful; all the more so if you can wear your success without flaunting it.

A charmed few achieve success apparently without trying but for most of us it is a struggle in which we must use all those other qualities this book discusses, especially motivation, stamina and integrity.

MENTAL AGILITY

Tell me where is fancy bred
Or in the heart or in the head?
William Shakespeare

Is it a coincidence that fitness and mental agility seem to go together? We think not. Physical fitness so often enhances mental agility. It may be for similar reasons that you feel better in a good-looking car or in a formal suit. If the trappings look good, they will give you a positive mental attitude – that business of self-image again. The fit body responds effortlessly to your mind's requirements – there is less of the time-wasting cranking up as your limbs move into action, less of a time lag between desiring and doing. In fact using a well-honed body paradoxically makes the body invisible; you no more need worry about whether it will obey your commands than you give thought to your heart beating regularly. With those physical doubts out of the way, you can concentrate your mind on what it does best – thinking, planning, analysing, and keeping a goal in mind.

But your subtle brain has its own maintenance problems – depressions, mental hang-ups, accustomed ways of working that tend to resist change, fears and uncertainties. Congratulations – you are a human being after all. Just remember that those mental problems are as real as any broken limb and their effects on performance may be much longer lasting than a broken bone. Plenty of men will not admit this to themselves; we hope we have shown you that to do so is not a weakness but is another kind of strength. Through the self-knowledge such episodes bring, you further enhance your quickness of mind.

Not that self-doubt is such a bad thing; it leads you to examine your motivation and analyse your desires before they lead to over-hasty action. We all differ in this; you may naturally be able to live with uncertainty or be naturally indecisive. Men will tend to gravitate to jobs which suit their personality and where their personality is an asset rather than a drawback. For similar reasons, you will tend to associate with people sharing your mental traits and mental agility – not to do so will lead you into embarrassment or boredom.

MOTIVATION

Fortunately it is not necessary to classify and analyse the many varieties of emotions, sentiments, moods, passions and hungers whose mention may answer the question 'why did you do it?'
Donald Davidson

You can do what you want
If you don't think you can't.
So don't think you can't if you can.
William Inge

The health hero might say: 'OK, so motivation moves in mysterious ways, but anyway, it's good to have it, and I've certainly got it in fistfuls.'

To be a man is to be wanting, planning and doing. Why this should be so is not always clear, when it may be much more desirable to rest in a chair, drink in hand. You, restless man, are reading this book because you want to change something about your life. You now realize that enjoying physical health can contribute to mental determination, by taking worries about stamina and physical ability out of your planning equation. You know that your fit body will do what you want it to do.

You will now understand that it is normal for your motives to be mixed, satisfying several needs at once such as self-esteem, money, power and attracting a woman. Understanding your motivation, as with so many other mental skills, can only be useful self-awareness. When you understand why you really want something, you are better placed to know if your goal is really so important to you. You may come to realize that you have been concealing or over-rating its true value to yourself, so that it may, on examination, prove to be a waste of effort for a false goal.

You probably already know that people who are highly motivated can waste energy in fruitless enterprises, causing resentment in others, whereas a period of thought before action would have channelled their motivation more effectively. For such reasons it is helpful to examine your own motivation from time to time. How much you do so is a personal matter and will be a reflection of your personality. It will impress others that you can not only perform a project but plan it too, thinking through ramifications and implications before they become obstacles. You are still a man of action but your moves are calculated and deliberate.

COMPETITIVENESS

We will now discuss in a little more detail the struggle for existence.
Charles Darwin

Survival of the fittest.
Herbert Spencer (supporter of Darwin)

The health hero might say: 'Sometimes you have to be ruthless. I would never be so sly as to stab someone in the back – I'd let them see me coming, stab them in the stomach and make a clean job of it.'

Though some wish it were otherwise, the world runs on competition – for resources, jobs, sexual partners, within organizations and between friends. Raw aggressive competition is generally frowned on by most mature societies, although even competition wearing a velvet glove may be brutally severe on your ego. The health hero enters the fray with self-awareness and without losing sight of basic human decencies. He knows that simply to get the better of someone, however satisfying in the short run, can be counterproductive to a long-term relationship.

The supplier who feels his prices are forever being cut back, the squash partner given no mercy, the girlfriend whose views are constantly belittled – such short-term victories eventually sour the relationship to the point of grudging resentment at best, and complete breakdown at worst. The health hero knows his goals, and is rightly determined to succeed, but his sensitivity and integrity prevent him pushing his advantage into an oppression. In return, he enjoys respect from those who recognize that his competitive skills are applied with regard for others' feelings.

There will be areas of life where competition is greater than in others; you will tend to self-select into those areas according to how well you can cope with the competition of others, who may treat you with less dignity than you yourself demonstrate. This is where physical fitness and mental stability become important buttresses to a life otherwise led at the edge of tolerance. With your self-awareness, you will be better placed to judge when the rewards of competition are no longer satisfying your deeper needs, so that a move towards a less harsh lifestyle is taken from informed choice rather than in a state of cynical burnout.

CONFIDENCE

Fortune favours the brave.
Terence

This can be interpreted as 'confidence is a sort of bravery'. The health hero might say: 'I trust my own judgements, but I listen to others; I have my own beliefs, but I respect others' beliefs; I am confident, but not over-confident.'

We recognize confidence in others often as much by what it is not, as by what it is. Confidence is not someone's belief that they are always right; not an inability or unwillingness to let others have their say; it is not belittling what others achieve nor is it constantly repeating previous successes. Such behaviour we regard not as confidence but as arrogance and self-importance. Confidence involves knowing when to press your point and when to allow others the advantage. It is a strength to recognize others' values, even when they clash with your own judgement.

Accompanying confidence is a physical presence and behaviour that reinforces your strength of mind. This will have elements of looking healthy, and of carrying yourself in a confident upright manner. It includes good grooming, which declares that you take a pride in your appearance and which may reflect an inner pride in arriving at thought-out conclusions and views. Your body language will be adding to your air of confidence, with eye contact that is embracing and not an aggressive stare, with calm movements, coherent speech, knowing when to talk and when to give others their turn.

In relationships with other men, you are confident that you remain masculine, competitive and action-oriented but without denying your softer sides of consideration and integrity. Women respond to your self-awareness which allows you to acknowledge your frailties and doubts without appearing weak or indecisive but instead sensitive and subtle.

Confident of your mental and physical strength, you have the self-assurance to dare to test your limits and to attempt new experiences – in work, at leisure and in relationships. When people who are confident fail, their failure is not as likely to become a source of amusement to others who take satisfaction from seeing pride conquered. Instead such failure is the stuff of human endeavour – calculated risks taken in full awareness of your capabilities, where failure engenders sympathy and success merits applause.

Others often believe that the confident person seems to make his own achievements. Really it is that they have a prepared mind, assured in its own capabilities with the bravery to try harder and to pursue opportunity with more eagerness.

WISDOM

A truly great man never puts away the simplicity of a child.
Chinese proverb

The health hero might say: 'Part of being wise is knowing when to hold silent...'

Wisdom may be expressed in a pithy comment, an extended article, an opinion, a gesture. The wise man is not necessarily totally original. In fact, his opinions may be quite commonplace, but stated with sufficient edge and insight to open a new perspective on the way the world is. By common consent, you cannot become wise without having self-knowledge and without pondering on the lessons that life teaches us about the human condition.

The wise man has used his sensitivity to understand human relationships and the factors which power human endeavour. Even while exercising his stamina, competitiveness and motivation he can stand back from himself to reflect on his own behaviour and what inspires him. This allows him to draw conclusions that others recognize for their truth and their comforting knowledge that we are not each entirely alone in our struggles.

Wisdom often starts with a deep understanding of your own work that allows you to move beyond the sheer mechanics of the job to deeper insights into your occupation. Where others remain engrossed in the day-to-day details of work, the wise man sees the philosophy behind the activity. This often cannot be expressed simply as facts but as an understanding of the tradition behind an activity. In the same way, the wise man reflects on his relationships and on the behaviour of society as a whole. With a rueful smile he accepts his mistakes as well as taking a justified pride in his abilities and attainments.

The wise man is deeply aware of his limitations as much as his capabilities. He has learnt to accept that there are some things he will never change nor achieve and to regard this with humility rather than resentment. He can look back at actions which may have been wrong or misguided, but which were driven by a sense of integrity from which he can take satisfaction.

His wisdom extends to his friends and colleagues; he understands that people are complex, their motivations rarely entirely rational and that inconsistencies are more likely due to chance than hypocrisy. Wisdom makes a man more tolerant of both himself and others. And often more humorous too. This is a generosity of spirit that makes the wise man attractive to men and women, while his own satisfaction is from a fulfilled and healthy life.

APPENDICES

1 Complementary therapies

The judicious use of complementary therapies can be of enormous benefit to well-being in its broadest interpretation – well-being of body, mind and spirit. Men tend to be more sceptical of the claims of complementary therapists and less willing to explore what is available than women. But for those who are interested, there follows a brief guide to some of the major therapies, listed in alphabetical order. Therapies which might be judged to be slightly fringe, even by the standards of complementary medicine (e.g. crystal healing and radionics) are not included.

Many natural medicines, such as herbal and homeopathic preparations and Bach Flower Remedies, are widely available through pharmacies and health stores. If you undertake self-treatment, remember the simple rule – if in doubt, don't. If you are uncertain about which remedy to take or in what dosage, or have any other questions, talk to a qualified practitioner. If you have any adverse reaction to a remedy, stop taking it at once, and seek professional advice. If you suffer from any underlying condition, or are on long-term medication, talk to your GP before taking complementary remedies. Similarly, if you consult a professional practitioner of complementary medicine, tell him or her about any orthodox drugs you are taking. Orthodox and complementary drugs can sometimes interfere with each other's actions. Proprietary natural medicines should not be used long-term – if symptoms persist, consult a qualified practitioner or your GP.

Word-of-mouth is often a good way to find a complementary practitioner – personal recommendation always inspires confidence. Check that your chosen practitioner is a member of a relevant regulatory body; this should guarantee that he or she has undergone appropriate training, including continuing professional training, has relevant insurance, accepts a code of ethics and is subject to disciplinary action if he or she breaks it. Any therapist should be willing to discuss the likely costs of treatment, and to set an acceptable, easily understood scale of fees. He or she should also be able to tell you how long it will be before you see significant improvement to your problem.

Most complementary therapists will offer general advice on diet and lifestyle, in line with the recommendations in Part One of this book. Many will stress the importance of becoming consciously aware of your breathing – knowing how to inhale and exhale fully. Becoming aware of your breathing, and breathing deeply and evenly whenever you have the opportunity, can bring enormous health benefits, largely through stress-reduction – but stop at once if you feel dizzy or light-headed. Many Eastern therapies assume that when we breathe in, we draw positive vital energy into our bodies, and when we breathe out we expel negative energy. The concept of vital energy is of importance in Western therapies too.

The therapies listed below all adhere to the principles of holism – that the body, mind, spirit and emotions are inter-dependent parts of an integrated organic whole – the whole you. Although most of them can treat the symptoms of disease on an ad hoc basis, most practitioners much prefer to think that they are tackling the underlying causes of dis-ease (the hyphen is important) in a systematic manner. Reputable therapists are unlikely to begin treatment without first building up a detailed picture of your unique constitution – your needs, aversions, desires and expectations.

Complementary therapies can be particularly useful for combating the stresses and strains of modern living, and many incorporate specific relaxation techniques. Learning a relaxation technique, preferably one that you can incorporate into your daily routine, can have a huge positive benefit on your health, perhaps lowering blood pressure, helping to regulate mood swings, or alleviating the effects of headaches. Of the therapies listed below Alexander Technique, aromatherapy, reflexology, massage, Bach Flower Remedies, T'ai chi and yoga are particularly helpful in promoting relaxation. In addition, you might consider meditation or visualization – contemplative techniques which can calm an overactive mind and promote a state of being where all the background chatter which normally fills our consciousness fades away. Or you might benefit from autogenic training – a gentle form of self-administered psychotherapy which teaches special mental exercises to help you relax mentally and physically. When it comes to relaxation and stress relief, never forget the importance of breathing.

ACUPUNCTURE

This originated in China, and involves using needles to stimulate points, called acupoints, on the body. It is believed that these points lie at significant junctions of energy lines, or meridians, which form a sort of map of the flow of vital energy through the body. Stimulating the acupoints is believed to balance or redirect the flow of vital energy. Acupuncture uses the body's own healing energy to prevent the onset of ill health in the first place and to revitalize those who feel generally under the weather or constantly tired. It is also an extremely effective method of pain relief, particularly for pain in the muscles and joints, and for headaches. A branch of acupuncture called auricular therapy, concerned solely with needling acupoints on the ears, can help those suffering from addictions, especially to alcohol or drugs. It can also lessen the effects of damage to the ears. Treatment produces sensations of warmth in the ear, and increases local blood circulation. Self-stimulation of the acupoints through gentle finger massage in a clockwise direction is called acupressure – it is particularly good for headaches.

ALEXANDER TECHNIQUE

This is a system of re-education that is aimed at helping us regain the natural balance, posture and ease of movement we had as children, and to eliminate learned habits of slouching or slumping. You are taught to become aware of how you are using your body and to think about new ways of keeping your spine free of tension. You are shown how to hold your head to minimize tension in the neck, and great emphasis is placed on breathing. The Alexander Technique can help with stress-related conditions, including constant tiredness and anxiety. It can also alleviate breathing disorders, and pain in the back, neck or joints. Sportsmen use the Technique to help them improve their co-ordination, and to apply their energy efficiently. Actors and singers use it not only to enhance their grace and poise, but also as a means of improving their powers of voice projection.

AROMATHERAPY

This is very popular among women, and there is no reason why men should not also benefit from aromatherapy. Aromatherapy uses oils extracted from aromatic plants, herbs and trees – for example lavender, rosemary, rose, ylang-ylang, and sandalwood – to promote both physical health, and emotional and spiritual peace. It is often used in conjunction with massage, when the physiological benefits of the massage reinforce the psychological benefits of the healing oil. Aromatherapy oils can be added to your bath, which is great for stress-reduction; used as inhalations (put two to four drops on your handkerchief and breathe in deeply) to relieve nasal congestion or the symptoms of colds and flu; or applied neat to the skin to help with problems such as athlete's foot, scabies and cold sores. Note that some oils should not be used neat, and before using oils in this way, conduct a simple skin test – add one drop of the relevant oil to one teaspoon of almond oil, rub the mixture on to the skin on the inside of your wrist and leave it unwashed and uncovered for twenty-four hours. If you suffer any sort of reaction, do not use the oil. Men with thinning hair or dandruff might be interested to know that essential oils can be used in shampoos to improve circulation in the scalp and to promote healthy hair growth. If you suffer from allergies or asthma, consult a qualified aromatherapist before using essential oils.

AYURVEDA

This is the name for the Indian science of life. Ayurveda, which is based on a complex underlying philosophy, is the traditional medicine still widely practised in India and Sri Lanka. Like Western orthodox medicine, it is a comprehensive health-care system. Ayurveda incorporates detoxification, diet, exercise, breathing, meditation, massage and herbs. Herbs are used both for detoxification and as part of remedies designed to correct different sorts of energy imbalance in the body – disease is believed to be a symptom of such imbalances, and an important aim of the skilled practitioner is to eliminate them. Yoga can be a significant part of ayurveda.

BACH FLOWER REMEDIES

These are another therapy popular with women, but which can also benefit men. There are thirty-eight different Bach Flower Remedies, all widely available in pharmacies and healthfood shops. Remedies are prepared by steeping flowers in water, which thus becomes energized with their energy print. The energy is then fixed by adding alcohol. The remedies are very good for healing and balancing negative emotional, spiritual or psychological states, such as fear, uncertainty, indecision and despondency. Busy executives, or men under any type of stress at work, could consider packing Bach Rescue Remedy in their briefcases – this combines the energy of several flowers and acts as a sort of cure-all, for a quick boost to mental or emotional well-being. (It also has physical effects, and can be used in first aid.) Bach Flower Remedies can help men suffering from a variety of sexual problems. Whether erectile dysfunction or ejaculation problems have a psychological or emotional component, the remedies can help. They also have a role in helping individuals, and couples, cope with the stress of sub-fertility.

CHIROPRACTIC

Many men who are otherwise sceptical about complementary therapies happily consult a chiropractor about back pain, perhaps resulting from a sports injury. Chiropractors work on the musculo-skeletal system – bones, muscles, ligaments and tendons, concentrating especially on the spine. Practitioners use a variety of manipulative techniques; direct thrusts using different parts of the hand and wrist are often used on joints in the neck or spine, and account for the loud popping noise sometimes heard during chiropractic manipulation (this is caused when gas bubbles in the fluid between joints burst). Alternatively joints may be gently stretched, using more indirect pressure. The practitioner will often use special manipulations to relax a muscle before making a joint adjustment. It can help neck, shoulder and back pain, and relieve headaches and many digestive problems.

HERBALISM (CHINESE)

Herbalism, together with acupuncture and T'ai chi, forms the basis of traditional Chinese medicine, a comprehensive system of health care still widely practised in Hong Kong and China. Herbs are used to prevent ill health, and to treat both mental and physical illness, and to balance emotional upset. Ginseng is a well-known Chinese remedy – it is used to stimulate flagging energy, including mental and sexual energy. Tiger balm is also widely available – it is used to relieve aches and pains. Proprietary remedies are available for many minor complaints, including colds and flu, respiratory illnesses and digestive disturbances.

HERBALISM (WESTERN)

Medicinal herbalism uses the curative properties of various parts of plants, such as flowers, trees, bark, nuts, seeds and herbs, both to maintain good health and to treat disease. Herbs can be taken in a variety of forms – tinctures, teas, infusions and decoctions, creams and ointments, capsules, etc. For the sportsman, hot or cold compresses steeped in an infusion of rosemary, for example, can help ease aches, pains and swollen joints. Echinacea is widely available in tablet form, and can help boost your immune system and ward off infection. Many plants can also help the insomniac, especially valerian and hops. Digestive problems frequently respond well to treatment; useful herbs include camomile, peppermint and ginger.

HOMOEOPATHY

The art of treating like with like, homoeopathy relies on the belief that a substance that causes particular symptoms can also be used to cure those same symptoms. For example, when we sting ourselves on a stinging nettle, our skin feels as if it is burning or scalding. Hence a homoeopath might prescribe the remedy urtica, which is derived from the stinging nettle, to treat conditions accompanied by burning or scalding sensations. Remedies are derived, via successive dilution in water and alcohol, from plant, mineral and animal sources – some from positively dangerous sources, such as tarentula, derived from the famous large black spider whose bite was said to cause dancing mania. By the rule of like cures like, tarentula is used to treat conditions characterized by frantic behaviour. Homoeopaths have a range of options when prescribing for the special problems of men – those affecting the penis, prostate, testicle and scrotum. The remedy selected will reflect your individual constitution.

HYPNOTHERAPY

In hypnotherapy, a hypnotherapist induces a light trance in the client. In this hypnotic state the client can do one of two things. He can either bring to consciousness repressed or hidden memories, thus conferring new forms of understanding that enable him to release the cause of persistent problems and move on in his life. Alternatively, he can become receptive to suggestions which will help him accept, or reject, patterns of belief or behaviour. Hypnotherapy can thus be a powerful aid for those fighting addictions to alcohol, cigarettes or drugs; and for those suffering traumas or phobias, such as fear of flying; and for those wanting to boost self-image and self-esteem. In unskilled hands, hypnotherapy could be potentially dangerous, so always choose a therapist very carefully.

IRIDOLOGY

This is a diagnostic therapy. An iridologist will examine the iris of your eye to determine the state of your health, and detect any potential physical or psychological problems. Your eyes will be examined with a small torch, or magnifying glass, and perhaps videoed, or photographed, allowing the practitioner to view them in detail.

The left iris relates to the left-hand side of the body, and the right iris to that on the right. Each part of the eye relates to a part of the body; spots of colour, the fibres of the iris and the position of marks are all significant. Colour gives a general indication of constitution: blue-eyed people have a tendency to develop arthritis and ulcers; brown-eyed people have a tendency towards atherosclerosis and gallbladder problems; green- or grey-eyed people have a tendency to digestive problems.

KINESIOLOGY

This is another diagnostic therapy. Kinesiology means the study of movement. Practitioners believe that they can learn about your physical, emotional and mental health by testing muscles. The system is used to detect and rectify niggling, sub-clinical health problems before they develop into major health problems. Practitioners believe that channels of energy course through our bodies. When we are healthy, energy flows freely, but when we are at risk of ill health, energy becomes blocked. The practitioner tests for blockages by isolating a given muscle, and then touching a point on the body connected to it by an energy channel, while at the same time exerting mild pressure on the muscle. If you can resist the pressure, your energy is flowing freely; if not, it is blocked.

KIRLIAN PHOTOGRAPHY

Also a diagnostic therapy. This is based on the theory that we are all electrical beings, and that electrical energy can be photographed and analysed. You will be asked to place your fingertips, toes, hands or feet on photographic plates, on a machine which emits a high-frequency electrical signal. The image produced gives an indication of the quality of your energy, which varies with health and mental state. Your energy pattern can give an early warning of the onset of disease, so that appropriate treatment can be given. Kirlian photography is not appropriate for those who wear pacemakers, or have metal pins in their bones (metal interferes with imaging).

MASSAGE

Most men would be delighted to receive a massage; it has well-known stress-relieving and relaxational effects. At its most basic, massage means the manipulation of the body's soft tissues with specific techniques, such as stroking, knuckling, pummelling or kneading. It is often combined with aromatherapy, and plays a big part in ayurveda. Various types of massage may be offered, including Swedish and shiatsu. Sometimes massage can be delivered via jets of high-pressure water. Sports massage is widely used to maintain sportsmen at a peak of physical fitness, and to alleviate the effects of injury.

NUTRITIONAL THERAPY

This uses diet and vitamin and mineral supplementation to balance the body and prevent illness. There are three basic diagnoses: food intolerance, nutritional deficiency and toxic overload. The most common food intolerances are to wheat, diary produce, nuts, eggs, yeast, shellfish, citrus fruits and artificial colourings. These are often detected via elimination diets – elimination programmes should not be undertaken without supervision. Nutritional deficiency is tested for using blood, sweat or hair analysis. Toxic overload is diagnosed through analysis of symptoms and lifestyle. Sometimes fasting, or juice fasting, is recommended.

OSTEOPATHY AND CRANIAL OSTEOPATHY

As with chiropractic, many men who are otherwise sceptical about complementary medicine are willing to try osteopathy, and its sister therapy, cranial osteopathy. Osteopaths do not concentrate on the spine as much as chiropractors and instead focus on releasing tension in tight muscles. They employ a variety of, mostly very gentle, techniques for achieving this. Cranial osteopaths use a particularly light touch to manipulate the bones of the skull. Osteopathy can help with sports injuries, repetitive strain disorder, arm and hand pain, and neck and back pain. Pain resulting from constant vibration, perhaps from a steering wheel if you drive miles each day, responds well. Cranial osteopathy can prove beneficial for those suffering from migraine or sinusitis.

REFLEXOLOGY

Practitioners believe that each part of the body is reflected on the feet, and that stimulation of the reflex points by specialized massage techniques can stimulate the body's natural ability to heal itself. Reflexology can be used preventatively and can greatly alleviate a range of stress-related conditions. Many reflexologists massage the feet in the following order: toes, reflecting the brain, face and sensory reflexes; inside edges, reflecting the spine; hollows beneath the balls of the feet, reflecting the solar plexus; the base of the toes, reflecting the neck and throat; the balls of the feet, reflecting the chest, heart and upper arms; the insteps, reflecting the digestive and urinary systems; and the heels, reflecting the pelvis and legs.

T'AI CHI

Many men enjoy T'ai chi, and practitioners can often be seen in city parks and other open spaces. T'ai chi is a gentle art, which has an important role in traditional Chinese medicine. It employs meditation and calm, smooth and sometimes very beautiful dance-like exercises to improve the health of body, mind and spirit. During T'ai chi exercises the practitioner becomes consciously aware of his breathing, and attempts to co-ordinate breathing with the movements. In order to make a significant difference to health, T'ai chi needs to be practised regularly – the art takes many years to master. Shortened versions of some of the longer traditional routines have been developed to fit in with busy Western lifestyles.

YOGA

Like T'ai chi, yoga pays great attention to breathing, and also incorporates meditation. Many of the poses have masculine names – like two of the balancing poses which are called the Eagle and the Warrior. Yoga is intimately linked with tantra. In tantra, physical exercises are used as a means of promoting an ecstatic (originally religious) experience. The use of sound, sight and light are all important, as is the sublimation achieved during sex. Tantric techniques can help a couple to find new depths of intimacy, openness, respect and meaning in their relationship, as well as having a marked impact on their physical lovemaking. Ejaculatory control is given particular prominence.

If you want further information about any of these therapies, or any not listed here, you could try contacting the Natural Medicines Society, an impartial organization which acts on behalf of consumers of natural medicine, as well as promoting research into the efficacy and safety of remedies and therapies, and also lobbies politicians on issues of importance to those who use natural medicines.

2 Useful addresses

Alcoholics Anonymous
PO Box 1
Stonebow House
Stonebow
York YO1 7NJ
Tel: 01904 644 026 (or see
local phone directory)

ASH (Action on Smoking
and Health)
16 Fitzhardinge Street
London W1H 9PL
Tel: 0171-224 0743

British Heart Foundation
(diet and general advice)
14 Fitzhardinge Street
London W1H 4DH
Tel: 0171-935 0185

CancerBACUP (cancer-
related matters)
3 Bath Place
Rivington Street
London EC2A 3JR
Tel: 0800 181 199

Council for Complementary
and Alternative Medicine
(general help on finding
accredited therapists)
179 Gloucester Place
London NW1 6DX
Tel: 0181-968 3862

CRUSE (advice and support
after bereavement)
Cruse House
126 Sheen Road
London TW9 1UR
Tel: 0181-940 4818 (or see local
phone directory)

Health Education Authority
(general advice on healthy
living, diet and exercise)
Trevelyan House
30 Great Peter Street
London SW1P 2HW
Tel: 0171-222 5300

ME Association
PO Box 8
Stanford-le-Hope
Essex SS17 8EX
Tel: 01375 642 466

MIND (National Association for
Mental Health)
Granta House
15–19 Broadway
Stratford
London E15 4BQ
Tel: 0181-522 1728
Information line: 0345 660 163

Natural Medicines Society
Market Chambers
13A Market Place
Heanor
Derbyshire
DE75 7AA
Tel: 01773 710002

Relate National Marriage
Guidance
Herbert Gray College
Little Church Street
Rugby
CV21 3AP
Tel: 01788 573241

The Samaritans (for those in
despair and with suicidal
thoughts)
Tel: 0345 90 90 90 (or see local
phone directory)
e-mail: jo@samaritans.org

Seasonal Affective Disorder
(SAD) Association
PO Box 989
Steyning BN44 3HG
Tel: 01903 814 942

The Sports Council (advice on
exercise, sport and taking it up)
16 Upper Woburn Place
London WC1H 0QP
Tel: 0171-273 1500

Books, videos and men's magazines are all good sources of information on a healthy lifestyle. Your local library should be able to make suggestions. Many organizations, such as Relate, publish books which are widely available through bookshops. It might be wise to invest in a good, all-round encyclopaedia for the lay man, e.g., *The Royal Society of Medicine Encyclopaedia of Family Health* (Bloomsbury). All the mainstream men's magazines – *Men's Health, Esquire, GQ* etc. – carry regular articles and advice on all the health-related topics covered in this book, and can provide welcome ideas and inspiration for the man who wishes to improve his well-being.

INDEX

balanitis 99
baldness 176–9
  causes 176–7
  theories of 178
  treatments 177–8
bathing 170
benzodiazepines 150
bereavement, as stress trigger 143
birth, presence at 115–17
blepharoplasty 184
blood pressure, checking 40
blood sugar levels 75
blood tests 43–4
  for life insurance 46
  PSA (prostate specific
  antigen) 40, 54
BO (body odour) 170
body hair, excess 179–80
body language 188
body mass index (BMI) 21
bone cancer 57
bowel cancer 56
  checking for 40
brain damage 47
brain tumours 64
breakfast 16, 19
breast cancer 55
breath, bad 170–1
breathing exercises 38
breathing patterns 42
British Heart Foundation 218
Brooke Advisory Centre 114
burnout 134–6
  symptoms 135
  theories of 135

caffeine addiction 158
calcium 15
calorie consumption 6, 8, 22

camomile 81, 141, 214
cancer
  bone 57
  bowel 40, 56
  breast 55
  gastrointestinal tract 56
  gullet 56
  Hodgkin's disease 57
  leukaemia 57
  lung 55
  lymphoma 57
  pancreas 56
  penis 67
  prostate 8, 53–4
  skin 57
  stomach 56
  testicular 6, 8, 40, 54–5
CancerBACUP 218
candida 168
carbohydrates 13, 23
cereal 16
CFS (chronic fatigue syndrome)
  76–7
chakra balancing 38
change, coping with 136–48
cheerfulness 160
chi kung 38
childlessness 119–20
chiropractic 63, 141, 213
chlamydia 6, 8, 96–7
cholesterol 16
  checking 40, 43
  and heart disease 52
chromium 15
chronic fatigue syndrome (CFS)
  76–7
cigarettes *see* smoking
circumcision 67–8
  women's attitude to 98

integrity 195–7
intercourse 90
    experimenting 101–2, 123
    see also sex
intrauterine contraceptive
    devices (IUCDs) 113–14
iridology 46, 215
iron 15
irritable bowel syndrome (IBS)
    73
IUCDs (intrauterine
    contraceptive devices)
    113–14

jargon 188
joint pain 63–4

kidney function
    testing 44
    urine tests 40
kinesiology 46, 215
kirlian photography 46, 216

lecithin 19
lethargy, natural remedy for 141
leukaemia 57
life insurance 45–6
    examination 45–6
    questionnaire 45
lifestyle, stress triggers 143
lifting 62
light pollution 37–8
lipid levels, testing 43
liver function, testing 43–4
longevity 198–9
lungs
    cancer 55
    protection 50
    testing 41–2

lymphoma 57

magnesium 15
male menopause 75–6
male psychology 132
manipulative therapy, for stress
    141
Marie Stopes Centre 114
marriage, as stress trigger 143
massage 38, 63, 141, 216
masturbation 125
ME (myalgic encephalomyelitis)
    76–7
ME Association 219
medical tests 40–5
    follow-up checks 44–5
    general assessment 41
    presentation of results 44
meditation 38, 148
melancholy, natural remedy for
    141
menopause, male 75–6
mental agility 201–2
mental health 131–60
    programme for change
    161–4
Mental Health Foundation 219
migraines 64–5
MIND (National Association for
    Mental Health) 219
minerals 13–15, 24
minoxidil 177
moles 66
money, stress triggers 142
motivation 202–3
moving house, as stress trigger
    143
muscle pain 63–4
muscles 26–7